5-

Dementia Beyond Disease

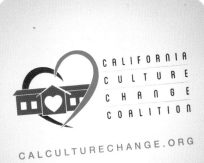

CALIFORNIA CULTURE CHANGE COALITION

CALCULTURECHANGE.ORG

Dementia Beyond Disease

ENHANCING WELL-BEING

by G. ALLEN POWER, M.D., FACP

Foreword by Richard Taylor, Ph.D.

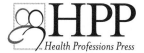

Baltimore • London • Sydney

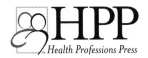

Health Professions Press, Inc.
Post Office Box 10624
Baltimore, Maryland 21285-0624

www.healthpropress.com

Interior and cover designs by Mindy Dunn.
Cover photo by Tracy Koflanovich. Copyright © 2014 by Tracy Jade Photography.
Cover photo taken at St. John's Penfield Green House homes.
Typeset by Barton Matheson Willse & Worthington, Baltimore, Maryland.
Manufactured in the United States of America by Versa Press, East Peoria, Illinois.

Quotes in chapters 4, 5, 8–10 from Shanks, L. K., *Your Name Is Hughes Hannibal Shanks:
A Caregiver's Guide to Alzheimer's*, copyright © 1999 by the University of Nebraska Press.

Chapter 3 epigraphs from John Lennon and Paul McCartney are lyrics from "I Am the Walrus"
and "Hello Goodbye," respectively. Both songs written by John Lennon and Paul McCartney.
Copyright © 1967 Sony/ATV Tunes LLC. All rights administered by Sony/ATV Music Publish-
ing LLC. All rights reserved. Used by permission.

The names of the people with dementia in this book have been changed to respect their privacy.

The information provided in this book is in no way meant to substitute for the advice or opinion
of a medical, legal, or other professional expert. This book is sold without warranties of any kind,
express or implied, and the publisher and authors disclaim any liability, loss, or damage caused by
the contents of this book.

Library of Congress Cataloging-in-Publication Data

Power, G. Allen, author.
    Dementia beyond disease : enhancing well-being / by G. Allen Power ; foreword by Richard
Taylor.
        p. ; cm.
    Includes bibliographical references and index.
    ISBN 978-1-938870-13-2 (pbk.)
    I. Title. [DNLM: 1. Dementia—therapy.   2. Dementia—psychology.   3. Health Services
for the Aged.   4. Patient-Centered Care.   5. Quality of Life—psychology. WM 220]
    RC521
    616.8'3—dc23
                                                                                    2014019016

British Library Cataloguing in Publication data are available from the British Library.

E-book edition: ISBN 978-1-938870-32-3

CONTENTS

ABOUT THE AUTHOR

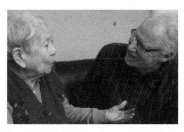

G. Allen Power, M.D., is a board-certified internist and geriatrician, and Clinical Associate Professor of Medicine at the University of Rochester, New York. A Certified Eden Alternative® Educator, Dr. Power is a member of The Eden Alternative board of directors and an international educator on transformational models of care for older adults, particularly those living with changing cognitive abilities.

His first book, *Dementia Beyond Drugs: Changing the Culture of Care*, won a 2010 Book of the Year Award from the *American Journal of Nursing*, and a 2011 Merit Award from the National Mature Media Awards. He was awarded a Bellagio Residency in Italy for April 2012 by the Rockefeller Foundation, during which he worked with Dr. Emi Kiyota on developing guidelines for sustainable communities that embrace people of all ages and abilities. In May 2013, Dr. Power was named one of "Five Leaders of Tomorrow" by *Long-Term Living Magazine*. He was interviewed for the film *Alive Inside,* winner of the Audience Award for Best U.S. Documentary at the 2014 Sundance Film Festival.

Dr. Power recorded introductory material for the U.S. Centers for Medicare and Medicaid Services (CMS) educational package "Hand in Hand," which is designed to help hands-on staff better care for people living with dementia. He also served on the technical advisory panel for CMS for their national antipsychotic drug reduction initiative.

Dr. Power serves in an advisory capacity for the Dementia Action Alliance, Dementia Care Australia, The South Africa Care Forum, Ibasho (Japan), and the Music and Memory project. He also serves on the Scientific Program Committee for Alzheimer's Disease International 2015 in Perth, Western Australia.

A trained musician and songwriter, Dr. Power has published three recordings, with songs performed by artists on three continents. Peter, Paul and Mary performed his song "If You Don't Mind," and Walter Cronkite used his song "I'll Love You Forever" in a 1995 *Cronkite Reports* documentary on the Discovery Channel.

FOREWORD

*Mighty oaks from little acorns grow.**

Hello, I am Richard Taylor, and for the past several, several years I have been living with the symptoms and diagnosis of "dementia, probably of the Alzheimer's type." Several years ago a youngish man (understand, I am 70 years old at this writing) called me and said he wanted to talk. That call from Al Power planted the acorn that has become the sapling that is now our on-growing relationship. We have spoken together many times, broken bread together many, many times, and conversed with each other for hundreds of hours.

I have self-discovered from him, and he from yours truly. Together we have each refined and expanded our own views of ourselves, of dementia, of aging, and of life in general. We have commiserated together about the awful state of affairs concerning dementia, stigmas, aging in this century, and living with the disabilities associated with dementia of this or that type. We have dreamt, plotted, planned, and wished what the future might look like, feel like, and be like for elders, folks who forget more than others, folks living in nursing homes, and folks whose brain functions have changed as they have aged.

We have both, from our own experiences, education, and perspectives, become advocates for a humane, humanizing understanding and response to aging. We both stand up and speak out most every chance we get about this increasingly clear vision we share of how the oaks should be shaped as they grow into the mighty classification. Concluding that the stigmas associated with the symptoms and label of dementia (I am fading away, I will die a shell of myself, I am more to be pitied than censured . . .) are reversible, we each in our own ways have become evangelists for a set of beliefs that is based on the fact that everyone is always a whole person until about 2 or 3 minutes after he or she has drawn a last breath.

This book is the second snapshot shown to the public of the work-in-progress that is Al's mind (the first being *Dementia Beyond Drugs* [2010]). This latest work is well worth your time reading and considering;

that is, how it might impact your relationships, your job, your family, and yourself. In these pages are the considered words of a considered human being. He has taken the original thinking of Abraham Maslow and updated, clarified, and focused the ideas and assumptions that we all share the same basic human needs and will share those needs regardless of what disabilities have befallen us. He makes a strong case for a major shift in how we view growing old in our society. He draws upon science, literature, and his own life experiences and thinking to suggest not just a better way to grow older, but the best (he would argue the only) way for individuals to grow into mighty oaks, regardless of soil conditions, droughts, insect and bacteria infestations, and dementia (pardon the mixed metaphor).

If you work with older folks, if you yourself plan on growing older, if you live with older folks, this is a challenging read. It offers the young and the not so young a vision of equality, purpose, and happiness for all of us as we grow old.

My hope is that reading this book will plant acorns in your own mind, from which mighty oaks will sprout. My hope is you, too, will become an advocate for the changes Al argues, reasons, and pleads for.

Join Al in his own journey of transformation from an overly educated acorn into one of the mighty oaks, a true believer in changing minds about people whose minds have been changed.

Richard Taylor, Ph.D.,
author of *Alzheimer's from the Inside Out* (2007)

---

*Mighty oaks from little acorns grow.

Meaning: Great things may come from small beginnings.

Origin: The word *acorn* does not come from *oak* and *corn*, as is popularly supposed, but from the Old English *aecern*, meaning berry or fruit. The tree genus Acer comes from the same root.

Before oaks were mighty they were first neither great, tall, or sturdy; or even just big. An example of an early variant of "mighty oaks from little acorns grow" is found in Geoffrey Chaucer's *Troilus and Criseyde* (1374): "as an ook cometh of a litel spyr" ["a spyr, or spire, is a sapling"].

The *Oxford Dictionary of Quotations* states that "great oaks from little acorns grow" is a fourteenth century proverb. Unfortunately, they do not include any details to support their view.

The "mighty" version is known, in the United States at least, from the middle of the nineteenth century. It appeared in A. B. Johnson's *The Philosophical Emperor: A Political Experiment* (1841). (http://www.phrases.org.uk/meanings/247100.html)

ACKNOWLEDGMENTS

"No man is an island." We are all guided and influenced by the wisdom and experience of those who walk beside us, and those who have gone before. Even "original" works reflect the influence of others, and the ideas set forth in this book are no exception. I have learned a great deal from countless conversations with the people I have met in my travels, and while I cannot possibly acknowledge every one, I would like to recognize a few of those individuals.

The seven domains of well-being that form the backbone of my approach are the result of a task force convened by The Eden Alternative®, which in 2005 produced a white paper authored by several specialists in transformational approaches to elder care. Those authors are: Nancy Fox, LaVrene Norton, Arthur Rashap, Joe Angelelli, Vivian Tellis-Nayak, Mary Tellis-Nayak, Leslie Grant, Sandy Ransom, Susan Dean, Suellen Beatty, Dawn Brostoski, and William Thomas. These seven domains provide a wonderful, value-based foundation for the framework I have created in this book, and I thank them for the inspiration. (Who says a committee cannot accomplish anything significant?) Thanks also to The Eden Alternative, Inc., for adopting and promulgating these domains in their Eden Alternative Domains of Well-Being™, and to Chris Perna, CEO of the Eden Alternative, for supporting and encouraging my use of them in creating the approach described in the book.

I am grateful to Health Professions Press, particularly Melissa Behm (President), Mary Magnus (Director of Publications), Julie Chávez (Sales & Brand Manager), Cecilia González (Production Manager), Diane Ersepke (copyeditor), Mindy Dunn (graphic, interior, and cover designer), and Kaitlin Konecke (Marketing Manager), for their ongoing support of my work and their creative input.

My heartfelt thanks to Richard Taylor for your wisdom and friendship, for the inspiring way in which you have lived, and your enduring sense of humor in the face of adversity.

Thanks as well to Christine Bryden for sharing another part of your story with me, and to all the people living with cognitive changes whose experiences continue to provide valuable instruction for those who will listen.

A huge thank you to Daniella Greenwood of Arcare Australia— for the operational initiatives you have shared, for your creative input throughout the book (from "word palettes" to "continual consent"), for your assistance with the framing of the first and last chapters, and for the brilliant pioneering work you do every day.

Many thanks also to Emi Kiyota for your guidance and input regarding the various aspects of environmental gerontology addressed herein. The Rockefeller Foundation funded the work that Emi and I did, through a 2012 Bellagio Residency, on innovative responses to global aging and the development of Ibasho Café principles (mentioned in Chapters 8 and 11). Thanks to Managing Director Rob Garris and the foundation for your support of that work.

In addition, a number of friends and colleagues have engaged in valuable conversations with me about various aspects of this book. Though I am bound to forget a few, I am especially indebted to Kris Angevine, Veronica Barber, Laura Beck, Jennifer Carson, Mimi Devinney, Carol Ende, Nancy Fox, Susan Frazier, Denise Hyde, Amy Mason, Kim McRae, Christa Merzeder, Kavan Peterson, Rebecca Priest, Peter Reed, Sarah Rowan, Nader Shabahangi, Bill Thomas, and, last in the alphabet but far from least, Carter Catlett Williams.

Thanks to Andrea Ruggieri for graphics assistance, to Joe LaMay for web assistance, and to Vicky Bournival for all kinds of assistance. Thank you to my colleagues during my years working at St. John's Home and St. John's Penfield Green Houses, for all you do every day.

Love and appreciation to my mother, Ora Power, for your inspiration and guidance, and as always, to my family: Eileen, Ian, Caitlin, (and now Aida too!), for your support and encouragement.

This book is dedicated to my parents,
Ora Babcock Power and the late George A. Power,
for all you have done through the years to provide
for our family's well-being.

Prologue

Read This First (and Last)!

My FIRST BOOK, *Dementia Beyond Drugs: Changing the Culture of Care* (Power, 2010), was an exercise in delayed gratification. It demanded a great deal of patience from the reader, as I slowly unwrapped an argument for a new approach to this constellation of experiences we have labeled "dementia." I even cautioned readers not to jump to the end to try and find the "answers." Some readers no doubt enthusiastically absorbed many of the suggestions in the last part of the book, but those who were able to remain "in the moment" tell me they found their rewards throughout.

This time around, I will not make you wait for the punch line. I have put it right here, at the top, so that even the casual reader will know where I am heading. This book discusses what I consider to be the central problem that plagues us in our work to create holistic, person-centered approaches, along with a new framework to help us move forward in the most successful way.

As I type these words, a vigorous debate rages over the proper way to respond to people living with dementia who exhibit various forms of distress. The frequent use of psychotropic drugs has been challenged—

1

first by a small but growing minority of authors and practitioners, and more recently fueled by increased media attention and government initiatives to reduce the use of such medications. Predictably, advocates of drug use are pushing back, and the debate rages on.

At one extreme are those who view dementia purely from a reductionist, biomedical perspective. This view holds that distress is the product of damaged brain cells and the chemical imbalances that result. They view such distress as "problem behaviors" and are quick to use such labels as "psychosis" to describe what they see. Drug therapy, including the use of antipsychotics, is a central part of their approach.

At the other end are the advocates of holistic, person-centered approaches. These disciples of the late Tom Kitwood, who have built upon the concepts he espoused in his seminal work, *Dementia Reconsidered* (Kitwood, 1997), look to unmet needs as a genesis for much of the distress we see. They believe that drugs are not the answer, and that distress should be met with an array of "nonpharmacological interventions."

In between these camps are the diplomatic "fence sitters," who allow that one should try nonpharmacological approaches first and foremost, with judicious use of psychotropic medications when the former are unsuccessful. The latter two groups compile algorithms and laundry lists of interventions that can be tried for a person who is distressed. Most of the available education on nonpharmacological approaches is centered on generating such lists and teaching how best to apply them.

In fact, all three camps are wrong. Or, if "wrong" is too strong a judgment, all three camps are addressing the wrong aspect of the situation. We have framed the debate around viewing distress as *the problem*, rather than as a symptom of something larger, and, therefore, the vast majority of our approaches are *reactive*, not *proactive*. This explains why no amount of medication, and no array of nonpharmacological interventions, serve to eliminate the distress experienced by most people who live with dementia. It explains why both the medications prescribed to "calm" people *and* the nondrug interventions that are designed to do the same need to be administered over and over, day after day, week after week.

Granted, there are times when a situation suddenly presents itself and some sort of response is needed. But that acute situation should not be seen as the problem, and the subsequent intervention should not frame the way in which we try to meet the person's needs over time, with or without the use of drugs. Let us take a look at each of the two approaches.

Pharmacological Approaches

In *Dementia Beyond Drugs*, I devoted a substantial chapter to critiquing the use of medications, particularly antipsychotic drugs, for the various expressions of need seen in people living with cognitive disabilities. In that chapter, I also challenged the design, execution, and analysis of the studies that purported to show a benefit of such medications and reviewed the emerging research showing the previously unrecognized dangers of these medications. I discussed the ways in which we improperly measure "improvement" and how we often make incorrect assumptions about cause and effect. Finally, the chapter concluded with a number of stories about the "awakenings" I witnessed when these medications were successfully withdrawn.

I will not revisit that very thorough discussion here. Suffice it to say that over the past few years since the book was written, further studies have strengthened those challenges and revealed these drugs to be even less effective and riskier than previously thought.

I make other observations about the drawbacks of drug therapy at various points in this book. These observations, however, build on a foundation set forth in my first book, and the reader who wishes to fully engage in these debates might wish to review that discussion (see Chapter 2, *Dementia Beyond Drugs*).

At this juncture, all I will add is that perhaps the greatest argument against the biomedical view that supports the use of such drugs is the multitude of cases in which a person's distress was solved through other approaches. These cases put the lie to the idea that we somehow needed to change that person's brain chemistry in order to relieve distress. Every time we see such a success, we should wonder how many other people's needs could be met without drugs, if we only could better identify the root causes.

Why Nonpharmacological
Interventions Do Not Work

This provocative heading may seem out of line for the author of a book called *Dementia Beyond Drugs*. Rest assured, I remain firmly rooted in the belief that most distress arises as expressions of unmet needs, and that drugs are not the answer. The problem lies not in that underlying

What Is Our Primary Goal?

All of the above suggests that, in spite of our efforts to reduce the use of potentially harmful medications, we are still not going about it the right way. Our federal government is right to be concerned about the overuse of such medications in people living with dementia, but a directive to reduce medication use by "X" percent by a given date (and the pledges of long-term care organizations to do so) puts the cart before the horse and sets us up for short-term gains that cannot be sustained over time.

In this book, I argue that although I am a strong supporter of reducing our reliance on psychotropic drugs, this is *not* our primary goal. It is a highly desirable outcome, but it is not the place to start. Furthermore, I do not even believe that reducing distress should be our primary goal. Once again, it is a very desirable long-term outcome, but distress is the "cough," not the "pneumonia."

I believe that our primary goal is to enhance *well-being*. This is a concept I discussed briefly in *Dementia Beyond Drugs*, but my subsequent work has convinced me that it is *the* central issue in improving the lives of people with dementia, and it provides the best vehicle for creating sustainable success.

In this book, I will expand on this primary goal of well-being to show how the concepts can be applied to the everyday lives of people with dementia, regardless of where they live or who provides their support.

I will present a framework for understanding well-being based on seven "domains": *identity, connectedness, security, autonomy, meaning, growth,* and *joy,* (Fox, et al., 2005). A chapter is devoted to each of the domains of well-being, and each is explored in a variety of ways. We will look at the universal features of each domain and the intrinsic and extrinsic factors that can threaten it for a person whose cognitive abilities are challenged.

The concept of "culture change" will again rear its head in this book, as we examine what needs to be done to *operationalize* this approach in various living environments. I will share many true stories that demonstrate the power of a well-being approach to greatly improve the lives of people who live with dementia, and their care partners as well.

I follow these chapters with a capstone chapter that demonstrates a radically different pathway to understanding distress and supporting the person. I will show how the well-being framework supports a new, strength-based approach—one that can produce more sustained success in reducing unnecessary medications than our usual "person-centered" approaches.

As with *Dementia Beyond Drugs*, the voices of people living with dementia (our "True Experts" and best teachers) will be heard throughout the text. Ignore them at your peril!

Finally, for those who want to take the full measure of this well-being perspective, I will digress here and there to explore concepts that are deeper, further out, or otherwise occupy a more challenging realm than much of our dialogue to date. No envelopes will remain unpushed.

Read on, and be well.

CHAPTER 1

A Brief History of the Experiential Model

Instead of thinking outside the box, get rid of the box.

—Deepak Chopra, M.D.

Listen:

Billy Pilgrim has come unstuck in time.

Billy has gone to sleep a senile widower and awakened on his wedding day. He has walked through a door in 1955 and come out another one in 1941. He has gone back through that door to find himself in 1963. He has seen his birth and death many times, he says, and pays random visits to all the events in between.

So BEGINS THE NARRATIVE of Kurt Vonnegut's acclaimed novel, *Slaughterhouse-Five* (Vonnegut, 1969, p. 23). This satirical fantasy tells the tale of an ordinary man, a World War II veteran, who was captured by the Germans and held prisoner during the 1945 allied firebombing of Dresden. Billy's later career as an optometrist is interrupted by an alien abduction, during which he is introduced to a race of beings ("Tralfamadorians") that gives him the ability to travel back and forth through time, revisiting various points of his life in a haphazard fashion.

A bit of an amateur time-traveler, Billy is occasionally able to use his gift as an escape from the more unpleasant periods of his life. But more often he finds himself bouncing back and forth through his life unexpectedly, reliving past traumas or other life events.

Like the aliens who abducted him, Billy comes to see all phases of his life simultaneously, such that the past and present often coexist in his mind. In fact, there are words and images that connect the past and present, and their appearance often pulls him out of the here and now to a faraway place, during which times people around him see him as being disconnected, or "zoned out."

Does any of this sound familiar? The previous paragraph might also describe a person living with one of the many conditions we collectively refer to as "dementia." In fact, it is an enjoyable exercise to reread this old classic in that way, imagining that rather than being whisked away to another planet, our hero instead begins to develop changes in his brain that pull him off the orderly path that leads most of us from past to future.

But such a path is not necessarily one of pure disability. It can also free the mind to see the world differently, and gain new ways to view the episodes of our lives. Vonnegut relates this philosophy while describing how the aliens read the chapters of their books:

> We Tralfamadorians read them all at once, not one after the other. There isn't any particular relationship between all the messages, except that the author has chosen them carefully, so that, when seen all at once, they produce an image of life that is beautiful and surprising and deep. There is no beginning, no middle, no end, no suspense, no moral, no causes, no effects. What we love in our books are the depths of many marvelous moments seen all at one time. (p. 88)

A similar view of the shifting of time can be found in Debra Dean's novel, *The Madonnas of Leningrad* (2007), in which the protagonist, Marina, a survivor of the siege of Leningrad, now lives with Alzheimer's in the northwestern United States:

> More distressing than the loss of words is the way that time contracts and fractures and drops her in unexpected places. (p. 96)

In time, Marina is also able to appreciate this transformation of time for its hidden gifts:

> For the moment, she forgets that she is lost, that she is weak and chilled and the soles of her feet are tender with sores. She pinches a leaf between her thumb and forefinger and holds it up. It is breathtakingly beautiful, the first new green of the world, the light of creation still shining inside it. She studies it. Time recedes, and she floats be-

yond it, absorbed totally and completely in this vision. Who knows how much time has passed? She is *beyond the tyranny of time*. Dmitri once left her sitting in a chair by the window and returned later to find her still entranced by the dance of dust motes caught in a shaft of late-afternoon sun. He claimed to have done three loads of wash in what felt to her like an instant. (p. 206, emphasis added)

Such exercises help us to reimagine the world of the person living with dementia. I have learned that deconstructing dementia in ways such as this can lead to new insights that were not apparent with the one-dimensional view that has dominated society over the last century.

My Personal Journey

In my own work, first as an internist in private practice and then as a geriatrician in long-term care settings, I became stuck in the traditional paradigm and fell prey to the same generalizations that have led us to stigmatize, disempower, and overmedicate millions of people across the United States and many more around the world. Eventually, I began to realize that my treatments were not changing the lives of the people in my care for the better; in fact, people often seemed worse off when these medications were prescribed.

I began to speak about nonpharmacological interventions, which would occasionally seem to help the situation, but eventually most people became distressed once again, and I found myself looking for another pill that might work better than the last. I also found myself in conflict, either with people who felt that drug use was necessary, or with people who supported other approaches in principle, but who just could not find the time and space within our rigid system of care to think and act differently.

Eventually, I drew two conclusions: (1) We need to change the way we look at dementia and the accompanying distress that people often experience, and (2) We need to transform the way we provide care, in order to support our new approach. But where do we begin?

The True Experts

It was at this time that I began to hear another group of voices—those of people who were living with the symptoms of dementia and who were writing about their experiences. Some, such as Dr. Richard Taylor from Houston and Australia's Christine Bryden, began speaking at conferences. I found myself fascinated—and often challenged—by what they had to say.

Over the past several years, I have come to view such people as the "True Experts" in dementia. I do not consider myself an expert; rather, I am a *professional student* of dementia. And with all due respect to my colleagues in neurology and psychiatry, they are not experts either, because this condition involves a change in our minds and, therefore, in the ways we see, hear, and think about the world around us. That is not something the rest of us can ever completely understand.

> We are expected to trust professionals who have not experienced our cognitive environment, and who were trained by others who have not experienced our cognitive environment. We are expected to trust them to do what is best for us. They believe they know not only what is best, but that they know *all* there is to know about how best to take care of us. (Taylor, 2011)

One of the biggest ways in which the True Experts helped me to move forward was to show me the degree to which they are stigmatized and silenced by even the most well-meaning people among us. True, the disabilities are real enough, but we are quick to assume that people's capabilities are less than they are, and we treat them accordingly. Kitwood (1997) referred to this as *positioning*.

How prevalent is positioning in our society? Much more than most of us realize. Consider the story of Ed Voris:

> In the book *Conversations with Ed* (Voris, Shabahangi, & Fox, 2009), Ed Voris discusses his life with Alzheimer's with Drs. Nader Shabahangi and Patrick Fox. With degrees in business administration and divinity, Ed worked in the affordable housing industry for many years. Shortly after retiring, he underwent a quadruple bypass operation, which led him to take stock and change gears, and he began working with people living with developmental disabilities.
>
> The earliest signs of a change in his thinking were much more apparent to Ed than to those around him. He began with some difficulties with word retrieval. Ed is extremely articulate, and so became highly aware when a word or phrase did not immediately come to mind. At times, he would have the rhythm of what he wanted to say, but the words did not follow. He also had a couple of episodes of losing his car in parking lots. We

have all had that experience, but Ed noticed that he was not as able to call up the sequence of parking as he had in the past to find his car.

So Ed went to his physician and requested cognitive testing. His eventual diagnosis of early-stage Alzheimer's first came to him via a three-page letter in the mail from his physician titled "Dementia," with further information enclosed. Not an auspicious start.

Ed went to his local Alzheimer's support chapter and other area venues in an effort to enlist additional resources and support, "and the uniform response was, 'Where is your family member or caregiver?' I had no authority of my own any longer" (p. 94).

At this point in time, Ed was living independently, driving, managing his affairs, and to those around him, speaking and functioning quite normally. But as soon as he mentioned the diagnosis, he was seen as incapable of processing information or acting on his own behalf. That is how quickly positioning happens. And this response came from people in organizations that are charged to support older adults and those living with dementia; people who would be expected to have the most training and sensitivity.

If our support organizations can be stigmatized in their outlook, how must the larger part of society view dementia? Ed's story also brings to mind an experience I had in the fall of 2012 while speaking at a conference with Dr. Richard Taylor.

Our host, Kim McRae, took us to dinner one night at a favorite local restaurant. A lovely woman greeted us warmly and chatted us up as we perused our menus. Richard was dressed elegantly, well groomed and charming as always.

The hostess asked us what brought us to town. When Richard told her our purpose, and that he had been living with dementia of the Alzheimer's type for several years, she was astounded. She repeated over and over that she could not believe he had Alzheimer's, asking how he could speak coherently and how could he go out to a restaurant to eat if he were afflicted with such a dreadful disease.

Richard kindly and patiently explained to her that many people living with the symptoms of dementia are able to continue to lead lives filled with engagement and purpose. I am not totally sure that she was convinced. She is not the first person to tell Richard he cannot possibly have had Alzheimer's all this time, because he "looks too good." Ed Voris has received similar comments from friends and acquaintances.

Having worked extensively with people who support those living with dementia, I can attest to the fact that these are all kind, caring people. Our problem is not so much one of character, but rather that we have a *paradigm*—a way of viewing dementia—that guides our attitudes and actions. Armed with this realization, I knew that, in order to build a new framework, I first needed to expose and remove the barriers created by the traditional approach.

The Biomedical Model as Cultural Hegemony

The term *cultural hegemony* comes from political discourse, and was often used in Marxist writings to describe the ways in which a ruling class exerts its own culture and beliefs upon the diverse members of society. It is a self-justifying process; although these beliefs and practices were put forth as being beneficial to all, they primarily benefited the rulers.

The medical profession, of which I am a proud member, holds high the ideal of doing what is best for the patient, and for the health of society. Unfortunately, acting from the position of "expert benefactor" can create a paternalistic approach to illness that produces a similar type of cultural hegemony. Such is the case of our traditional approach to dementia.

This traditional approach is what I usually refer to as the "biomedical model of dementia." Over the last several decades, we have come to view dementia as a constellation of degenerative diseases of the brain that are largely progressive, irreversible, and ultimately fatal. Our view focuses heavily on the deficits and losses experienced by those who live with dementia, and our policies emphasize the costs and burdens of the illness—on families, care systems, and society as a whole. We direct billions of funds each year to drug research and speak extensively about "finding the cure."

Please understand that there is nothing inherently wrong about this view. While some authors (e.g., Whitehouse & George, 2008) have argued that dementia may be less a disease than an extreme end of the spectrum of brain aging, the deficits and costs are real enough either way. However, the biomedical view of dementia is very *narrow* in its scope and, therefore, leads to a series of decisions and beliefs, from the bedside to national policy discussions, that diminish the very people we are trying to help.

Here is some of the "fallout" that results from a narrow biomedical view:

1.   Our deficit-based view of dementia leads us to characterize people purely in terms of those losses. They become "victims" or "dementia sufferers," and we use descriptive phrases such as "the long goodbye" and "the living death," thereby dehumanizing people in the process.

2.   This view leads us to create institutional, disease-based approaches to care. We practice "dementia care," create "dementia programming," or design "dementia units," rather than recognize people's unique histories and needs.

3.   A focus on deficits makes us quick to position people as being incapable and thus to disempower them, as in the case of Ed Voris. An important consequence of this positioning is that *our research ignores or discounts the subjective experience of people living with dementia.* This not only blinds us to new understandings of the causes of distress, but also leads us to incorrectly label many expressions as "psychotic" or "delusional."

4.   We view distress primarily as a function of diseased brain cells and chemical imbalances, and, as a result, we look almost exclusively to drug therapy to try and provide well-being.

This list raises another point that is often overlooked in our media coverage of federal nursing home initiatives: *Overmedication of people with dementia is not simply a problem in nursing homes; it is a community-wide problem that reflects broad societal views.*

Antipsychotic Use in Community-Based Living

Just how extensive a problem is antipsychotic use in the community? We do not have much data, because use of antipsychotic drugs for dementia is considered off-label, and there are no mechanisms for tracking these demographics as there are in nursing homes. The best we can do at this point is to study representative groups of community-dwelling adults and try to generalize the data to the larger population.

A study by Rhee, Csernansky, Emanuel, Chang, and Shega (2011) looked at a group of 307 people with dementia in the community who had been part of an aging study from 2002 to 2004. Of these, 19.1% were taking an antipsychotic drug. An additional 29.1% were taking antidepressants; nearly 19% more were either on medications for anxiety or antiseizure medications that are often used to stabilize mood. The sample was small, however, and not ethnically or geographically diverse.

Fick, Kolanowski, and Waller (2007) studied 959 people living with dementia in the southeastern United States and found that 27% were taking antipsychotics. And, as I reported in *Dementia Beyond Drugs*, my own survey of people moving into St. John's Home in Rochester in 2007, stratified by Mini-Mental State Examination score, showed that for those with an MMSE score of 10/30 or less, 50% had been taking antipsychotic drugs in their homes before moving to the nursing home.

Taken as a whole, these percentages may seem lower than the approximately 30%–35% of people with a diagnosis of dementia who receive antipsychotics in U.S. nursing homes. But considering the fact that at least four out of five people with dementia are living in the community, these studies suggest that the *absolute number* of people using antipsychotics is actually significantly greater in the community than in nursing homes. Extrapolating these data, it appears that the total number of Americans with dementia who are taking these drugs could be a million community-dwelling adults or more, compared to about 350,000 in skilled care settings. So if we are upset with antipsychotic use in nursing homes, we must first take a long, hard look in the mirror. Nursing homes are simply a reflection of a paradigm we all share.

Science and Public Policy as Casualties of Cultural Hegemony

It seems that all we talk about nowadays is the "search for the cure." To use baseball parlance, we put most of our resources into "hitting it out of the ballpark," and it is a huge ballpark—one whose home run fence is not even within our sight. We forget that you can also score points by simply advancing in small measurable amounts. If you put all of your energy into the elusive cure, you are bound to ignore the needs of today for millions of people with dementia and their care partners.

Every new angle of research, from mice to men, warrants news headlines as the "next possible breakthrough in the war on dementia." More press means more funding, so it becomes as much a public relations contest as a race to make true progress. I have had a number of interviews with prominent news media, but most of my words never saw the light of day. Why? Because I talked about ways to improve well-being and care. Not newsworthy.

The media want to talk about one of two things in relation to dementia: (1) how badly we drug people, and (2) who is leading the race to find new drugs. Does that sound like contradictory thinking? At first blush, you might say, "Well, no; looking for disease-modifying drugs is different from simply giving people antipsychotics." But both trends come back to the narrow biomedical view that the only path to a life worth living is through the pill bottle.

Ironically, among the biggest casualties of all of this are the very tenets of empirical science. Here are two examples of how scientific rigor can get lost in the shuffle:

1. Recent data from a Rotterdam study showed an overall 25% decline in the incidence of new cases of dementia diagnosed between 2000 and 2005, compared with a similar study conducted from 1990 to 1995 (Schrjvers et al., 2012). The result was widely circulated, and the media quoted the study team as saying, "Although the differences were nonsignificant, our study suggests that dementia incidence has decreased."

   No, with all due respect, your study does not suggest that. I know it looks that way, and it is perfectly believable, if for no other reason than due to our advances in cardiovascular health. But the study results were "nonsignificant." This means that, mathematically speaking, the difference in numbers is more likely due to chance than to a true reduction.

   Personally, I believe that the passage of time *will* show further decreases in the incidence of new cases of dementia that will reach levels of statistical significance. But until they do, we cannot jump to conclusions that are unsupported by the basic laws of research science, and it is irresponsible to report them to the world as scientific fact.

2. A study published in the *New England Journal of Medicine* followed a group of people living with dementia in nursing homes who were taking the antipsychotic drug risperidone (Devanand et al., 2012). They were randomized into two groups, and half had their drug withdrawn. However, unlike other, more carefully planned withdrawal trials (e.g., Fossey et al., 2006, and Ballard et al., 2008), no attempts were made to identify people's unmet needs or to provide any other approach to care in the study group. Their drugs

were simply and summarily stopped and replaced with a placebo.

Guess what happened? The people whose drugs were withdrawn had a higher rate of distress than those who were kept on the medication. Given the sedating nature of these drugs, this result is unsurprising; in fact, it should have been a foregone conclusion. Unfortunately, the authors not only missed a key intervention that would have helped their subjects successfully withdraw from the pills, they also used this flawed premise to reach a flawed conclusion: that the results of the study supported the use of antipsychotics.

Another way to view the second study is to suppose I had a hundred subjects and every day I would hit each of them on the head with a hammer and then give them a pain pill. If I took the pain pills away from half of the subjects, their pain would no doubt get worse. Does that prove that we should just keep giving everyone the pain pills? How about if we stop hitting them on the head?

To be fair, the *New England Journal of Medicine* study was valuable in that it taught one very important lesson that should not be ignored: If we simply stop these medications and do not do anything else, we are not meeting people's needs, and their distress will continue. This supports my contention in the Prologue that reduction of psychotropic drugs is not our *primary* goal. If we set drug reduction goals without first establishing a pathway toward better identifying and meeting people's needs, then we will ultimately fail to sustain those results, and, like the authors of the study, we will erroneously conclude that the pills are needed after all.

In fact, the title of the article also reveals the extent of biomedical thinking in this field of research ("Relapse Risk after Discontinuation of Risperidone in Alzheimer's Disease"). By using the term *relapse* to characterize the worsening of distress, the authors are suggesting that they felt the people on the drug had been successfully treated before withdrawal. Unless they had evidence that the elders were more alert, relaxed, and engaged while on the medication (which has *never* been proven using positive end points), chances are they confused sedation with effectiveness.

A New Definition of Dementia

Armed with these insights, any new framework for viewing dementia must first deconstruct the preconceptions of our traditional biomedical view and start with a clean slate. We must find a way to describe the process of cognitive change that is as free of judgment and stigma as possible, so that we can be open to new approaches and new solutions. In short, *we need to change our minds about people whose minds have changed*.

This was the thinking that led me to a new definition of dementia: *Dementia is a shift in the way a person experiences the world around her/him*. This is as neutral and generic a description as one can imagine. For many, it may seem too vague to be of use. In fact, if researchers were trying to find a new drug to slow the changes seen in the brain, then this definition would not contain enough information to guide them. But for the rest of us—those who wish to support people living with dementia—this definition is exactly what the doctor ordered for a better approach to life and care.

For the rest of us, the research definitions have led us astray, because the more we focus on tangled neurons, amyloid plaques, and tau proteins, the less we are able to see the *person* surrounding them. We focus on the pathology and respond accordingly. We lament the millions of neurons lost to dementia and ignore the many millions that work perfectly well. And we pin all of our hopes on the next pill, putting millions of lives on hold while we wait for that discovery that may or may not be coming next week, next year, or maybe not at all.

The fact is that changing our approach can produce more well-being for people living with dementia than any pill that is available today, or is likely to be available in the foreseeable future. Why? To put it simply, because well-being cannot be bottled.

For the rest of us outside the drug research laboratories, the *experiential* definition of dementia stated above is a better solution. While it may seem inexact, it is not the detail that is important, but rather the *mindset* that the definition provides. This mindset is what leads us to new answers, and a new paradigm for care.

The first advantage of this new definition is that it is one that connects, rather than separates us. Everyone reading this book has had a shift in the way he or she experiences the world, due to the life-changing experiences of aging, learning, and growth. This knowledge that our perspective can change as we go through life enables us to better enter the world of persons living with dementia and appreciate how they might view the world differently. This is a critical step in finding new solutions.

A second advantage is that this definition helps keep our focus on the whole person, rather than merely a disease process. It can help us to appreciate the words of Richard Taylor (2011) when he stated, "I am not *dying* of a fatal disease; I am *living* with a chronic disability."

Dementia as a Chronic Disability

In fact, seeing dementia as a disability (or changing ability) rather than a fatal disease creates a host of insights to which the biomedical view has blinded us. We see that people with dementia continue to learn new information, incorporate data, and use problem-solving skills to adapt to their changing perceptions. This encourages strength-based approaches to care.

A "different ability" view also helps us to see how we are failing to meet the needs of people living with dementia, and how we can begin to do better. I often ask my audiences to imagine a man without dementia whose legs have become paralyzed due to an injury, and who now needs a wheelchair. This is also a person whose experience of the world has changed quite dramatically. If such a person tried to enter a public building and encountered a flight of stairs, he would be stuck; but thanks to our disability laws, we have built ramps and other forms of assistance to remove the barriers caused by the disability. Why? Because we want people who are unable to walk to continue to succeed in a world of people who are able to walk.

However, in our biomedical approach, we have failed to build ramps for people with dementia. In this case, I am not referring to physical ramps so much as "cognitive ramps"—ways of helping a person whose brain is changing better connect to the world around her. Instead, we create living environments based on our view of the world, our daily needs, and our staffing patterns, and expect people whose brains are changing to adapt to them. And when they cannot, we diagnose a "behavior problem" and medicate them.

Imagine a doctor and nurse walking up to the man in the wheelchair as he sits at the foot of a large stairway. Imagine them saying to him, "We walk up the steps, so we'd like you to do that as well." And with much encouragement, they lift him out of the chair and lean him forward. What will happen? He will fall to the ground, of course, because his legs do not work the way they used to. And if he becomes angry with them for tossing him to the ground, it would be pretty silly for the doctor to say, "Well, he certainly has a behavior problem; let's give him an antipsychotic and see if it calms him down."

That sounds laughable, and yet, *we do this every day, in all living environments, for people with dementia.* We put them into situations where they cannot succeed, and then medicate the (entirely predictable) result.

The Experiential Shift

An experiential approach moves us from pills to ramps. It also incorporates the person's subjective experience to guide us in finding those ramps, rather than simply ignoring him because "he's confused."

> In the world of 19th century physics, most of the laws of the known universe were quantifiable; time and space seemed to be constant. Then in 1905, a relatively unknown patent clerk named Albert Einstein wrote a paper, in which he said, in effect, "Well, that depends." Exactly where an object was going and how fast was dependent on the perspective of the observer. If you and I are in two different circumstances, the laws might not apply equally. And if you were able to travel fast enough to approach the speed of light, even time itself could be bent or stretched.
>
> In publishing his paper, Einstein's theory of relativity challenged how we viewed the very nature of the physical universe. Here is my point: if time and space can actually change depending on one's perspective, what does that say about the way we judge the perceptions of people living with dementia?
>
> We are quick to judge whether or not a person is "oriented to place and time"; and if her reality does not match ours, we may label her confused or even delusional. But is it delusion, or is it "relativity"—processing input from the world around you, through the lens of a brain whose perception of the world is "in motion"?

The experiential view changes us in other ways as well. When we realize that changing experience is an integral part of life, we begin to accept this reality and stop trying to change the person into someone she can no longer be, as surely as we can no longer be our younger selves. At the 2011 "A Changing Melody" conference in Toronto (a wonderful event planned and executed in collaboration with people living with dementia), I met Jim Mann from Vancouver, who lives with

Alzheimer's disease. He explained it to me this way: "My life is not what it used to be; I have to accept that there's a 'new normal.'"

This is not an argument to end drug research. Accepting the "new normal" does not mean that we stop looking for ways to slow the progression of disability. But it keeps our research a bit more grounded in setting achievable goals.

So we are back to the main theme of this book, which is about finding the pathway to well-being. Although some readers may consider an experiential approach to be rather unscientific, in fact, it leads us to look at a lot of the "science" of dementia research and point out that, all too often, "the Emperor has no clothes." The experiential model detailed in this book leads us to challenge those traditional approaches to care that have long been accepted and implemented, but have never truly improved people's lives. It helps us to better hear the words and understand the needs of people living with dementia. It is a blueprint for the construction of ramps to continued well-being despite changing abilities. And it changes how we view our own mission as care partners in this important work.

In other words, an experiential view changes everything.

CHAPTER 2

The What and Why of Well-Being

He who lives in harmony with himself lives in harmony
with the universe.

—Marcus Aurelius

The part can never be well unless the whole is well.

—Plato

What's invisible to us is also crucial for our own well-being.

—Jeanette Winterson

WELL-BEING IS A CONCEPT that is difficult to pin down. There is no
single accepted definition. Indeed, many believe that well-being can
only be determined by each individual for him- or herself. "Hard to
define" means even harder to measure. The term includes the word *being*, and Thomas (2004) reminds us that, "To *be* is to create and sustain
relationships with the invisible and the intangible" (p. 118).

So how is it possible to construct a theory, not to mention a framework for supporting people, around such a vague concept? Are we left
to regard well-being the same way that former Supreme Court Justice
Potter Stewart regarded pornography ("I know it when I see it.")? Not
necessarily.

Despite the many varied interpretations of well-being, there are
common threads. From these threads, it is possible to create a theory
of well-being that can be applied in real-life situations and produce

measurable results. But in order to do so, we need to shift some more paradigms.

Traditional measures of "quality of life" and "quality of care" have arisen from our focus on biomedical approaches to care, and they reflect our own perspective as adults who continue to focus primarily on *doing* instead of *being*. The result is that we measure the quality of life and care for elders in general (and those living with dementia in particular) with scales that favor (1) medical outcomes, and (2) higher levels of functional and cognitive ability.

These are not bad outcomes to measure. They are important to all of us. But just like the biomedical view of dementia, they are limited and do not define the whole person. Imagine a person living in a nursing home that puts all of its effort into optimizing these traditional quality indicators. She might receive all of her medications exactly as prescribed, on time, without error. She might never fall, develop a bladder infection, or be physically restrained. She might receive all the required nutrition and calories and never go too long without being offered food. She might live her life without the discomfort and indignity of a catheter, a stool impaction, or a pressure sore. And yet, she might still hate her life and wish she were dead.

In fact, this is the experience of many people in long-term care environments, and many more living in the community. I do not believe that most people fear nursing homes because they feel they will not receive adequate medical and nursing care. Their fear comes from the loss of other important aspects of a life worth living that are too often left at the door. What is missing is what I am calling *well-being*.

Choosing Domains of Well-Being

During the past two decades, numerous authors have described schematics or models that identify elements, sometimes called indicators or domains, of well-being. In 2005, a taskforce of experts in transformational care (Fox, Norton, Rashap, Angelelli, Tellis-Nayak (V.), Tellis-Nayak (M.), Grant, Ransom, Dean, Beatty, Brostoski, & Thomas) was brought together by The Eden Alternative®, a nonprofit organization dedicated to improving the lives of elders and their care partners in all living environments. This group produced a white paper that challenged traditional quality-of-life measurements and instead offered seven domains of well-being: *identity, growth, autonomy, security, con-*

nectedness, meaning, and *joy* (available at http://actionpact.com/site/ culture_change_in_practice). The Eden Alternative subsequently expanded upon the original publication (Fox et al., 2005) in a 2012 white paper titled "The Eden Alternative Domains of Well-Being™: Revolutionizing the Experience of Home by Bringing Well-Being to Life" (available at www.edenalt.org).

One of the reasons I like this list is because these seven domains reject our tendency to define quality of life in terms of presence or absence of medical illness, or as a measure of our functional or cognitive abilities (i.e., what we can or cannot *do*). By contrast, these seven domains can exist independent of those factors. This removes the stigma of seeing a person with dementia as incapable of achieving well-being and gives us a strong directive to fulfill these needs throughout everyone's life. Indeed, these domains can be applied to any human condition, including terminal illness.

Really? Any Condition??

In 2012, as an Eden Alternative Educator, I was facilitating a workshop for 50 participants from Laguna Honda Hospital and Rehab in San Francisco. When I introduced these domains of well-being, a nurse practitioner asked a very challenging question: "I can see this concept applying to most people, but how about someone whose dementia is so severe that she is akin to being in a persistent vegetative state, or otherwise unable to communicate? How can we possibly support these domains in someone like that?"

Tough question. I paused for a moment to consider the question and collect my thoughts. However, before I could form a reply, a nursing assistant's hand shot up from the other side of the room. I called on her and listened as she taught the rest of the class and me how it was possible.

Her aunt was living in the nursing home and completely unable to engage or communicate with family or staff. Without batting an eye, the participant rattled off each domain of well-being and told us how the family was working to preserve it. Through a multitude of actions, from personalizing the room to sharing favorite music, flowers, memories, or prayers, the family engaged all of her senses to touch, kiss, sing, laugh, and connect. Since then, I have been convinced that these domains of well-being are truly universal.

This story also illustrates another important point. Kitwood (1997) wrote that personhood is an intrinsic quality, but it also implies recognition by others. Although the domains of well-being can be eroded by the disabilities of dementia, they can be supported and rejuvenated through the efforts of care partners. Indeed, it is incumbent upon us to place the support of well-being at the forefront of our goals in caring for people living with dementia. This goal never fades; in fact, it is arguably even more important as one's abilities decline.

In this book, I resequence the original Fox et al. (2005) list of domains and dedicate a chapter to each in the following order: *identity, connectedness, security, autonomy, meaning, growth, and joy* (Figure 1). Doing so creates a flow that I think will best educate and challenge the reader. It also suggests a framework through which we can enhance well-being for people living with dementia. I will demonstrate the power of this framework using the seven domains of well-being described above; however, I have designed this approach in a way that enables it to be used with other definitions as well (a few of which are described below).

There are many alternate views of well-being—far too many to list here. I will, however, mention a few, starting with Tom Kitwood.

Other Models for Well-Being

Kitwood has published two different schematics that revolve around the concept of well-being, though in slightly different ways than the domains I am using. Kitwood and Bredin (1992) published a list of 12 indicators of well-being. These are signs that a person has a positive sense of well-being and include such observations as helpfulness, initiation of social contact, and affectional warmth. However, these are not domains of well-being in themselves, and one could argue that not all people living with dementia can accomplish all 12, as some of them (such as the preceding examples) require the ability to "do" certain tasks.

Identity
Connectedness
Security
Autonomy
Meaning
Growth
Joy

Figure 1. A resequencing of the original Fox et al. (2005) domains of well-being reflects how each domain supports the next.

Kitwood and Bredin went on to say that these 12 signs indicate the presence of four, deeper "global states"; these come closer to the Fox et al. (2005) definition of well-being. The four global states are *sense of personal worth* (which I believe is comprised within the domains of identity and meaning), *sense of agency* (autonomy), *social confidence* (security and connectedness), and *hope* (meaning, growth, and joy).

In *Dementia Reconsidered*, Kitwood (1997) used the graphic of a flower to illustrate six "main psychological needs" of the person with dementia. The five petals of the flower represent *comfort, attachment, inclusion, occupation,* and *identity.* He reserved the center of the blossom for the sixth psychological need, *love.*

There are many parallels here with the Fox et al. (2005) domains of well-being. Both physical and psychological comfort are expressed largely in terms of security; attachment and inclusion comprise the important relationships seen in the domain of connectedness. Occupation refers to engagement in activity that has personal significance and is highly correlated to the domain of meaning. Identity is identical in both models. Finally, Kitwood saw love as the "all-encompassing need" (p. 81), which is served by the other five. In this way, it parallels the domain of joy, which I see as largely arising from optimizing the other domains.

Love is not exactly the same as joy, and the most common critique I receive when speaking about the Fox et al. (2005) domains is that love should be added to the list. There is a subtle difference in the lists, however. Love is a psychological need; it is not the same as a domain of well-being. Love can lead to joy, so they are connected in that manner. A reading of the domains listed by Fox et al. suggests to me that love is not a stand-alone domain, but rather a pathway to creating joy (as well as connectedness, security, meaning, and growth). Similarly, Kitwood's other psychological needs serve the Fox et al. (2005) well-being domains (except that *identity* works as both a domain and a psychological need). So they are not contradictory or exclusionary. Instead, they complement each other—one (Kitwood) being more of a list of processes, while the other (Fox et al., 2005) is more a list of outcomes.

Jane Verity (a former student of Kitwood and founder of the award-winning *Spark of Life* approach of Dementia Care Australia) has regrouped Kitwood's concept into "five universal emotional needs": *to feel needed and useful, to give care to others, to love and be loved, to have the power to choose,* and *to have one's self-esteem boosted* (Verity & Lee, 2008). Once again, these are presented as psychological needs and have much resonance with the seven domains of well-being.

Another popular approach to supporting people living with dementia is the Senses framework (Nolan, Brown, Davies, Nolan, & Keady, 2006). This approach emphasizes the primacy of relationships and encourages care partners to work to create a sense of security, belonging, continuity, purpose, achievement, and significance. Again, there is a great deal of overlap with the seven domains: security is equivalent; belonging and continuity align with aspects of connectedness; purpose, achievement, and significance all connect with meaning and growth; and significance aligns with identity as well. Autonomy and joy are less clearly represented with counterparts in this model.

A somewhat different way to look at universal needs is through the work of Carboni (1990), who compared the experience of institutionalized elders to that of our homeless population. From this, she developed seven attributes of "home": *identity, connectedness, lived space, privacy, power/autonomy, safety/predictability,* and *journeying.* She contrasted these with seven opposing attributes of "homelessness."

Once again, there are several direct correlations with the Fox et al. (2005) domains of well-being. Journeying contains elements of meaning and growth. Lived space could be seen as a function of identity, while privacy is a component of security. There is no direct correlate to joy in this model.

The Chilean economist Manfred Max-Neef pioneered a concept of nine fundamental human needs that he described as applicable across all cultures and all periods of human history. He believed that these needs were mutually interactive, not ordered as Abraham Maslow theorized with his own "hierarchy of needs" (Maslow, 1943). The nine fundamental human needs identified by Max-Neef and his colleagues are: *subsistence, protection, affection, understanding, participation, leisure, creation, identity,* and *freedom* (Max-Neef, Elizalde, & Hopenhayn, 1991). Leisure (occasionally translated as "idleness" in English renditions of his work) is an interesting concept that Max-Neef added after his original eight needs were published, and ties in nicely to the concept underlying the next model to be described.

MAREP Living and Celebrating Life through Leisure Project

One could argue that *all* of these models are not quite adequate, because they represent substituted judgment of what others need; in particular, none of these was developed with the input of people living with dementia. But thanks to the work of the Murray Alzheimer Research and Education Program (MAREP), we have some guidance here.

MAREP represents a collaborative project, along with researchers from the University of Waterloo, Ontario, Canada, and people living with dementia. Through regular meetings, people living with dementia help set agendas for research and education priorities, even producing educational materials with a series of *By Us, For Us*© guides (see Chapter 7). MAREP also produced a conference titled A Changing Melody, which ran for 5 successive years and opened the 2011 Alzheimer's Disease International conference in Toronto.

One of the concepts being developed by the researchers at University of Waterloo is a shift away from the traditional long-term care practice of programmed activities toward a more individualized celebration of leisure experiences. In creating a tool for determining individuals' preferences, 200 people living with dementia were interviewed about what aspects of these experiences they considered most important. The results were tabulated and the group combined them into seven areas: *being me, being with, finding balance, seeking freedom, making a difference, growing and developing,* and *having fun* (DuPuis, Whyte, Carson, et al., 2012).

In Figure 2, I have taken some liberty with the sequence of the seven areas in order to highlight how well these align with the Fox et al. (2005) domains of well-being. They are virtually identical, the only possible exception being "finding balance," which I have placed next to "security." However, security for people living with dementia is largely a matter of finding balances: between privacy and socialization,

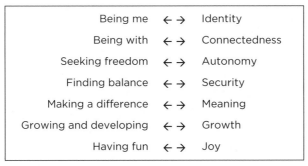

Figure 2. Alignment of the Fox et al. (2005) domains of well-being with the MAREP meaningful leisure experiences.

spontaneity and predictability, safety and quality of life, and so on. We will expand on these concepts in Chapter 5.

The bottom line is that, regardless of how one defines well-being, the framework I present in this book can help us support people living with dementia in any environment, provided it fulfills certain criteria: (1) we must be able to make the case that our domains are universal, or nearly so, across most ages and cultures; (2) the domains should be attainable to some degree, regardless of one's underlying medical condition and cognitive/functional status; and (3) when the domains cannot be preserved by the person alone, other care partners should be able to help maintain them.

The Fox et al. (2005) domains of well-being fit these criteria very well, and it is especially gratifying that they are also supported in principle by the people living with dementia who were surveyed by MAREP, and, therefore, provide an excellent framework to combine with the experiential model (Power, 2010). If there are other domains you prefer, they will likely be applicable in the same manner. I invite you to follow along with this list of seven, and we will develop tools that you should be able to apply successfully to whatever definition of well-being works best for you.

Each of the next seven chapters will be devoted to one domain of well-being. As promised in the Prologue, we will explore each domain fully in order to identify our ultimate goals in supporting people with dementia, understand why some approaches work and others fall short, and dig much deeper than much of the literature on person-centered care has explored to date. In doing so, each domain will be presented on a continuum along which we can begin to travel; a pathway toward a life worth living for all.

Transformational Models of Care—A Brief Refresher

As with *Dementia Beyond Drugs*, this book will weave concepts with recommendations for transforming the care environment, a process commonly referred to in long-term care circles as "culture change." In my mind, the greatest shortcoming of the available literature on person-centered approaches to dementia care has been the relative lack of ink devoted to this topic. It is simply not sufficient to discuss new approaches to supporting people living with dementia without including a discussion of transforming the care environment. Here's why.

No matter what new philosophy of care you adopt, if you try to bring that philosophy into an institution, the institution will kill it, every time. In this case, "institution" refers not so much to a physical structure as to a mindset. Even so, the institutional mindset is as rigid and unyielding as any brick-and-mortar stronghold, and is fortified by operations and processes that have been bolstered by time and repetition. These reinforced attitudes and behaviors do not melt away overnight. If we want a new idea to take hold, we have to find ways to shift our operations to support this new way of thinking and ingrain it into the fabric of daily life. That process is what we call "culture change."

In formal long-term care settings, this involves a total revamping of any aspects that support old ways of thinking and prevent new ones from taking hold. In this respect, we talk about three types of transformation: *physical, operational,* and *personal* (Power, 2010).

Physical transformation means creating structural environments that support the values of home and the domains of well-being, rather than supporting institutional ways of providing care in the narrow biomedical sense. Personal transformation comprises both *intrapersonal* components (how we view dementia and people who live with dementia), and *interpersonal* components (how we interact with and support them).

Operational transformation acts as a lynchpin for the other two, because neither a homey physical environment nor a holistic mindset is sufficient unless we support them through our daily actions and interactions. This is more than simply changing job titles or redrawing the organizational chart. It involves a variety of daily processes, such as how decisions are made (and who has input in those decisions), how information is communicated, how conflicts are resolved, and how domains of well-being are supported for the people who live *and* work there. It even goes as far as to transform job descriptions, policies and procedures, and performance evaluations.

This last point is critical because, as Upton Sinclair once wrote, "It is difficult to get a man to understand something, when his salary depends on his not understanding it!" (Sinclair, 1935, p. 109). For example, if an organization makes a point of saying that employees should value relationships over tasks, but if the evaluations (and pay raises) still measure performance that is based primarily on task completion, one can predict where the employee will devote the most attention.

Another important consideration for long-term care is that culture change is for everyone involved in the system—not just providers and community members, but also regulators, legislators, insurers, and reimbursement mechanisms. The organizations' paychecks are no less incentive based than those of their individual employees. They will devote their resources to the areas that are rewarded by our reimbursement system and our annual surveys. If those systems reward tasks and interventions over humanized care, we cannot expect providers to change their approach. Members of *every* stakeholder group need to begin a deep process of self-evaluation and determine how they themselves need to grow in order to best support the work of others.

The following chapters will not confine themselves to life in the nursing home, however. Just as our biomedical approach and overuse of psychotropic medications reflect societal attitudes and patterns, so too can people with dementia suffer the plagues of institutionalization in community settings, including their own homes. This may not be so obvious to those who look through a biomedical lens or are overly focused on the physical surroundings of the nursing home; but when looking through experiential eyes and focusing on domains of well-being, it becomes apparent that a person living at home can have an existence that feels just as institutional as in any nursing home you can imagine.

So while some readers were not able to easily translate the lessons of *Dementia Beyond Drugs* to community living, our focus on well-being in this book will make the concepts much easier to understand and apply across the entire continuum of living environments.

A Final Word about Terminology

As with *Dementia Beyond Drugs*, I am making an intentional effort to shift my language, and I invite all readers to do the same, because our word choices often frame our attitudes. I will continue to point out some of these shifts as they occur, though many others were already described and defined in *Dementia Beyond Drugs*. However, I would like to make a few comments about the words we have used to describe our overall approach.

Up to this point, I have used the common phrase of *person-centered care*, a term coined by Kitwood and popularized by the many people who have built on his holistic, individualized approach. For many other people, however, the language has evolved further since its introduction in 1997.

Many practitioners of culture change, including Eden Alternative advocates, have used the term *person-directed care* instead. The rationale is that many people have claimed to be person-centered, but in fact have acted very paternalistically toward the people in their care, making choices that they think are best for the person, with little or no input from the person. Saying "person-directed" is a way of raising the bar by insisting that a concerted effort be made to solicit the person's own direction, or if the person is unable, to solicit the direction of a person who knows him well and can best represent his interests.

Others have proposed the term *relationship-centered care*, suggesting that the best care comes primarily within the context of meaningful relationships, rather than simple advocacy on the part of individuals. While meaningful relationships are valued in all similar philosophies, this approach uses the terminology to keep those knowing relationships in the forefront.

My personal feeling is that any of these terms can be perfectly correct or can be misused if viewed too narrowly—the real key is how they are applied. For example, it is perfectly fine to say, "I am person-centered," as long as I recognize that I should strive to have a knowing relationship with the person and solicit meaningful direction from the person as well.

So while I tend to be a stickler about many word choices, this is one area in which I am willing to pay less scrutiny to the actual words, and more to the *intent* behind them. DuPuis, Gillies, Carson, et al. (2012) have taken this a step further by suggesting that our goal is to develop *authentic partnerships* with people who live with dementia. In my mind, this may be the best choice of all, and one that I have been using more and more in my own speaking and writing. This term nicely encompasses both concepts of self-direction and relationship. It also removes the word *care*, which is problematic in that many people equate care with medical and nursing interventions, rather than considering a more holistic relationship, or simply living life itself.

The Eden Alternative® redefines care as "helping another to grow." I like this definition, but it often requires some explanation to people who have long been taught to see care as treatment. For that reason, I would recommend that those who wish to keep their "person-centered," "person-directed," or "relationship-centered" language consider replacing the word *care* with *living*.

Lastly, as with *Dementia Beyond Drugs*, I alternate the use of male and female pronouns when used nonspecifically, rather than defaulting exclusively to the male gender. I also use pseudonyms for the people living with dementia whose stories have not been publically shared.

Now, let us explore the path to well-being, one domain at a time. As you will see in the next chapters, each of the seven "definitions" of the domains of well-being (Fox et al., 2005) is actually a list of several features that make up the domain. This is not simply a concession to many different interpretations of each domain, but rather an acknowledgment that each domain has many facets that must be recognized in order to fully realize one's potential for well-being.

Each of the next seven chapters will follow a similar outline, although each chapter will also contain unique elements and digressions, as the spirit moves. Each chapter begins with a discussion of how the domain of well-being can become especially challenged in people who live with the symptoms of dementia. In each case, we will examine both *intrinsic* and *extrinsic* factors that erode the domain of well-being. And in each case, we will show how the extrinsic factors produce *excess disability* that can equal or even surpass the effects of the brain changes. In addition to examining long-term care environments, we will also explore the ways in which well-being can be challenged in home and community-based living.

In *Dementia Beyond Drugs*, I included a "modest proposal" to eliminate segregated living (so-called memory care housing or special care units) for people with dementia, and I predicted that it would be the most controversial topic in that rather challenging book. In my travels since the book was published, I can say that the prediction was correct. I will also say, however, that, although I felt like a bit of a pariah at the outset, I find the idea gaining support over time, much like Juror #8 (Henry Fonda) found in the film *Twelve Angry Men*. I am hoping the day will come when we find the "defendant" with dementia "not guilty" and set her free to live in the larger community.

In my initial argument, I listed several clinical, operational, and ethical reasons for my opinion; I will not repeat them here. But my conviction remains strong in this regard, so I will face the doubters and take my argument further in this book. Each chapter contains a brief section detailing how a segregated living environment can erode that particular well-being domain.

Many people who disagree with this opinion are currently working in such environments. Often, I think they are offended by this opinion, feeling that it does not recognize the value of the care and support they provide. Let me state unequivocally that this has nothing to do with the compassionate, talented *people* who provide care in such settings. Many such places provide top-notch care within that format. My criticism lies with the "dementia unit" paradigm and operational format; in culture change the message always revolves around the system and the mindset, not the wonderful people who do such work.

Finally, each chapter concludes with suggestions on how we can use the three dimensions of transformation—personal, operational, and physical—to help restore each domain of well-being, even for those who are far along the path of forgetfulness. These closing sections are then used as a template in Chapter 10 to design a powerful tool for decoding distress and providing a path to living a fuller life, free of potentially harmful psychoactive drugs.

Let us begin where any person-centered approach should begin, with the domain of identity.

CHAPTER 3

Identity

I am he as you are he as you are me and we are all together.

—John Lennon

Hello, hello, I don't know why you say goodbye, I say hello.

—Paul McCartney

The most beautiful sound in the world is the sound of my own name.

—Ed Voris

LENNON AND MCCARTNEY WERE an interesting study in identity. As the primary songwriters of The Beatles, they simply put both of their names on all of their song copyrights, even though most of the songs were written primarily by one or the other. And yet ardent Beatles fans can usually identify the originator of each song, due to each individual style and voice. "Yesterday" is classic Paul; "Across the Universe," classic John.

We continue to see the individuals inside iconic groups such as The Beatles. But when we superimpose a different label, such as "Alzheimer's" or "dementia," the individuals begin to disappear in our minds.

Lennon's quote above, taken from the enigmatic song "I Am the Walrus," reminds me of the way we tend to lump people together based on their diagnosis, and lose our perspective of the person as a unique individual. McCartney's line from "Hello Goodbye" brings to mind the common image of the person with dementia as "fading away." (Cathie Borrie deserves credit for this song connection, as she often uses it to introduce oral presentations of her book, *The Long Hello*

[Borrie, 2010], a brilliant and moving portrayal of her relationship with her mother, who lived with Alzheimer's.) I address both of these preconceptions in this chapter. The third quote, from Ed Voris, who is living with Alzheimer's, reminds us of the intrinsic beauty we attach to our own identity and our struggle to preserve it.

Identity Defined

Fox et al. (2005) describe identity as *being well-known; having personhood; individuality; wholeness; having a history.* Just as I rearranged the sequence of the well-being domains, I also find it useful to examine these facets of identity in a somewhat different order. I begin with *personhood*, which speaks to the heart of Tom Kitwood's work.

Kitwood (1997) describes personhood within the context of social dynamics, as "a standing or status that is bestowed upon one human being, by others, in the context of relationship and social being. It implies recognition, respect, and trust" (p. 8). So, in one sense, those around you must recognize your identity for it to be complete. But he also declared that "being-in-itself is sacred" (p. 8), implying that personhood also has an intrinsic aspect and exists even when not appreciated by one's social network.

The terms *individuality* and *wholeness* suggest two different but complementary aspects of identity. *Individuality* means that each person remains a unique individual, despite changing cognitive abilities. *Wholeness* goes further to mean that the person remains whole, despite changing cognitive abilities. Both of these words directly challenge the dominant paradigm for viewing dementia.

> I am not half full. I am not half empty. I am a whole person and will continue to be a whole person until I draw my last breath. (Taylor, 2011)

Finally, "being well known" and "having a history" refer to the fact that one's individuality also results from a multitude of unique life experiences. This suggests that fully understanding a person's history is an important key to helping the person maintain identity.

How Dementia Challenges Identity

In this and the next six chapters, I examine the well-being domains in relation to the intrinsic and extrinsic challenges to each. The brain changes associated with dementia can create *intrinsic* challenges to each domain of well-being. In addition, certain features of one's living environment, common stigmas surrounding the person, and our approaches to care can create *extrinsic* challenges that further complicate the situation.

Intrinsic Challenges

From the standpoint of the intrinsic changes associated with the condition, the primary challenge to identity comes from forgetfulness. The lost access to memories makes it difficult for a person to construct and maintain the various aspects of her personal history that form her identity.

We define our own identity in many ways—by our occupation, cultural background, relationships, multiple roles within the family, standing within the community, political leanings, or spirituality. As these details become harder to recall, we can feel incomplete, set adrift from the attachments to which we have been so firmly anchored throughout life. This can lead to an existential crisis and fuel much of the grief that people experience, particularly in the earlier stages of forgetfulness when a closer proximity to the details of memories lost creates a more acute sense of grief.

One such example is the book *Losing My Mind* (DeBaggio, 2002), in which the author writes of his experience with Alzheimer's. Though eloquently written, the author's narrative is heavily laden with anticipatory grief:

> One part of my life is over. A new unknown life begins today, a kind of death march, although one we all take at one time or another. There are more mysteries than ever at a time when knowledge should have provided almost enough. For me, now, my focus is on the cemetery. The only question is how many months or years before I move in. (p. 45)

Extrinsic Challenges

Dealing with these losses is difficult enough, but society's values and perspectives create an external view of a person living with dementia that erodes identity even more acutely. This plays out in a multitude of ways. I described much of this negative effect in Chapter 1 as "fallout from the biomedical view of dementia." Examining this in more detail, our view of a person living with dementia as an empty-headed, tragic "victim" creates a lack of appreciation for the individual and his intact strengths and abilities, and also perpetuates the stigmas that rob him of the wholeness and personhood necessary to preserve identity. He becomes less than human in our eyes.

These stigmatized images run the gamut from piteous to repulsive. Behuniak (2011) examines the common view of people with Alzheimer's as "zombies." She postulates, "It is this politics of revulsion and fear that directly infuses the discourse about (Alzheimer's disease) and shapes it" (p. 72). She argues that, while the brain changes are real enough, there is also a very real social construct around this negative stereotype that colors our dialogues about care, support, and allotment of resources.

Behuniak goes on to state that three of the distinguishing characteristics of the zombie that are classically portrayed in Hollywood films, "[A]ppearance, loss of self, and loss of the ability to recognize others," reflect a common view of people living with Alzheimer's (p. 78). Therefore, when we lose sight of people's identity, we can lose sight of their humanity, and equate them with "the living dead."

Is the stigma really that bad? The article cites a study by Aquilina and Hughes (2006), which compares quotes about people with dementia with descriptions of zombies and finds that they are largely indistinguishable. Behuniak warns that such a comparable view harms people with dementia because it is "at odds with the notion of death with dignity or, to be more accurate, life with dignity" (p. 86). And buried within this perception of lost humanity lies a powerful tool for disempowering and disenfranchising the person, even at the earliest onset of cognitive disability. (We will explore this further in Chapter 6, "Autonomy.")

Edvardsson, Winblad, and Sandman (2008) echo the perils of losing a life with dignity with this warning: "If staff believe that a diagnosis of [Alzheimer's disease] means that personhood is gradually being lost and that there is nothing left of the person, the ethical demand to take care of these people, who have placed their trust in them, disappears because the person has gone anyway" (p. 362). We see this concept played out in countless *self-fulfilling prophecies*, a term applied by Lyman back in 1989. I expand upon this throughout the book. Examples of this attitude are commonly seen in statements such as, "Move him to the dementia unit—they won't care if someone comes into their room naked." Or, "There is no need to use consistent staff for her baths—she won't remember them anyway."

At "A Changing Melody 2011," a conference in Toronto, Christine Bryden identified the "stereotype of dementia" as the cause of both stigma (for society) and fear (for the person living with the condition):

> What is the cause of the stigma and fear? It's the stereotype of dementia: someone who cannot understand, remembers nothing, and is unaware of what is happening around them. This stereotype tugs at the heartstrings and loosens the purse strings, so is used in seeking funds for research, support, and services. It's a Catch-22, because Alzheimer's associations promote our image as non-persons, and make the stigma worse. (Bryden, 2011)

Larry Rose (2003) describes his own experience with stigma and fear this way:

> I thought when I got the diagnosis, that I would die before I made it home from the Doctor's office. Or, in the alternative, be in the nursing home within a week or so. Such was the stereotype [sic] Alzheimer's patient that I had seen on TV. (p. 48)

For most of us, the ultimate loss of identity is death, so we equate the changes of dementia with a continuous or recurrent death. Even without succumbing to the zombie image, we too often embrace stigmatized descriptions of dementia as "the long goodbye" or "fading away."

In the video, *20 Questions, 100 Answers, 6 Perspectives* (Brilliant Image Productions, 2012), Dr. Richard Taylor describes the negative effects of this view, not only on the person with dementia, but also on those who care for him:

> I think other people, and sometimes ourselves, see us as "fading away." And in fact, they even call it "The Long Goodbye." . . . And so I believe people don't come around to see you as much as they used to. And they don't because who wants to say "goodbye" every day, maybe for 10 years? I never said "goodbye" to you in the sense that I thought you were dying, until you were diagnosed. . . .
>
> People say to us we're going to die twice: we're going to die as ourselves, and then we're going to die as somebody that nobody knows. I don't believe this helps anyone, seeing people this way, thinking about them, and especially telling them; telling them with your eyes, telling them with your hugs, and telling them with behaviors that you used to perform, and that you don't anymore, because it's just so painful to see you fading away. I think it's at the root of

most of the sadness, most of the stress that's in the hearts of caregivers, because someone they love is "fading away"; they are dying right before their eyes.

This perfectly captures the grief that the loss of identity visits upon both people with dementia and their care partners. In a shared memoir of her husband's experience with Alzheimer's (Simpson & Simpson, 1999), Anne Simpson feels her husband's anticipatory grief as well:

What I can't begin to fathom is the pain it must cause him to know he will have to give up reading! This disease doesn't just mean gradually losing things. It also means anticipating losses, going through long periods of mourning before the final separation. Then anticipating another . . . and another. (p. 40)

But many people have acquired a special type of wisdom that comes from living with dementia. They have come to see their lives as far from over, for they have had to deal more directly and personally with grief, loss, and the sense of impending death. They have had to ask themselves, "Who am I now?" (and, as Christine Bryden titled her first book, *Who Will I Be When I Die?* [re-released in 2012]). Often they discover a revived sense of identity—one that adds "dementia" to the résumé, but includes a whole person nonetheless. As Anne Simpson's husband, Robert, observes later in their memoir:

We're still here. We still have ideas and can express them. Just be patient and listen to us. We are real people! There is a difference between the people and the disease. The disease is what makes us different. (p. 52)

So when we get too lost in grief over our loved ones, Richard Taylor shakes us like a 1950s movie doctor telling a histrionic patient to "Get a hold of yourself!" He reminds us, "One of my crusades is to say, 'I'm still here, dammit!' . . . and the fact that I am saying 'I'm *still* here' is probably wrong—I *am* here!" (Brilliant Image Productions, 2012). The lesson: Preserve identity, celebrate personhood, and create meaning in the moment.

Such lessons are hard to embrace, however, when societal attitudes continue to bombard us with the stigmas, which are not simply individual biases; they are institutionalized and embedded in our systems of care. This brings us back to the opening quote from "I Am the Walrus." Individual identity becomes lost in a sea of generalities about "dementia patients"; we see the disease instead of the person, and we treat him accordingly.

The medical community has reinforced such biases through their use of standardized cognitive tests. Although such tests often give useful clues to specific areas of disability or to overall levels of function, focusing excessively on them erodes identity by reducing a person to a series of discrete cognitive tasks. In hearing about Ed Voris's frustrations with such cognitive testing approaches (Voris, Shabahangi, & Fox, 2009), Dr. Patrick Fox observes that "The kind of process you (Ed) went through decontextualizes the person as a social being and places him or her in a clinical setting that is controlled by a system of thought" (p. 46).

The identified deficits then become the basis for wholesale judgments about a person's capabilities, ignoring the fact that many complex and integrative tasks remain well preserved. (We will explore this further in Chapter 6.) In long-term care, this plays out in such scenarios as talking over a person to a co-worker during a meal, speaking about someone as if she were not there, or even holding meetings about her care without including her. We also see it in activity programming, which traditionally has been driven by the use of standardized cognitive assessments that measure deficits in discrete areas of thinking and match them with prescribed, disease stage–specific activities (see Chapter 7).

Many other operational and structural decisions in long-term care are made on the basis of this homogenized, deficit-based view of dementia. One of the most prevalent examples is the ever-more-popular segregated living area.

Segregated Living and Identity

I have had several discussions with caring people who explain why they think their segregated living environments are better. The argument often sounds like this: "In our experience, we have found that *they* respond well to 'x,' that *they* respond poorly to 'y,' and that *they* like (this or that aspect of the environment)." In other words, the main arguments for segregated living revolve around a set of generalizations and stereotypes—individual identity is lost.

The homogenization of meaningful engagement in long-term care is something that plays out repeatedly in segregated living areas. Because the living space is created around a disease instead of a group of unique individuals, life and care revolve around that disease-based view. This homogenization occurs not only with activity programming, but also with care plans, meals, and other aspects of daily life.

The problem with a disease-based approach to care is that it squelches identity and is too often blind to the uniqueness of the individual. When a community is defined by a disease (or even more so by a single stage of the disease), this creates a setting where the opposite of individualized care often results.

The other major argument I hear for segregation is that this type of arrangement greatly reduces the work demands on the staff; it is felt that there are fewer variations in the type of approach and activities they need to employ when people have a similar cognitive level. But, once again, this is an overgeneralization that ignores the maxim that "If you've seen one person with dementia, you've seen one person with dementia." While caring for people with dementia is admittedly very hard work, homogenizing life and care in an effort to ease the workload erodes identity.

Let me acknowledge that a few segregated communities have produced some outstanding results. One example is the work that has been done at Beatitudes Campus (which includes a community for people with dementia in Phoenix, Arizona) to eliminate the phenomenon of "sundown syndrome" (Power, 2012a).

The staff at Beatitudes realized that much of the late-day restlessness and distress that our biomedical model blames on a damaged brain is actually more a function of environmental factors, which I see in terms of damaged *identity*. "Sundowning" often reflects people with unique and changing biorhythms being forced into a rigid, institutional pattern, thereby causing their bodies to rebel. It can also reflect the reawakening of old patterns of activity from a person's prior job or past leisure activities and is often cued by the commotion of people donning coats and saying "goodbye" at the change of a shift.

Beatitudes has all but eliminated this so-called sundown syndrome for over a decade by putting an end to the late-day commotion and by instituting a policy of "rest as needed" that listens to the individual's rhythm, rather than an artificial schedule of rest and activity. In other words, they have restored one aspect of identity by following the individual's lead, and have eliminated sights and sounds that might lead to other aspects of one's past history arising out of context.

This is a spectacular achievement, but I do not feel it invalidates my point about segregated living. Why? Because those same operational changes can be applied just as easily and effectively in integrated living areas. There is nothing about the Beatitudes solution that demanded a dementia-specific environment in order to succeed. We may assume that people without dementia are immune to change-of-shift commotion and institutional schedules, but they are not. This is a solution that can work for everyone.

Physical Aspects of Segregated Living

Many of the physical trappings of segregated environments also revolve around claims that they are better for "dementia care." I have not found this to be a valid argument either. An example of this is a study of environmental enhancements designed to help support the various disabilities associated with dementia (Zeisel et al., 2003). This study employed eight design principles, ranging from privacy and personalization of living space to access to outdoor paths and gardens to an overall homier and less-institutional environment. The study was well designed and demonstrated improvements in various types of distress as a result of the modifications.

Once again, the modifications described in this study have great validity and are clearly effective in improving well-being, but almost all of the features described are ones that all of us would want, with or without dementia. The few features that might be specifically more helpful to a person living with dementia (such as various wayfinding cues) could easily be incorporated into any integrated living area. The advantage of a more "universal design" approach is that those people without dementia who subsequently develop different levels of forgetfulness can age in place and not have to move to another, better designed living area.

In fact, a widely touted set of design principles for dementia-specific living (Calkins & Sloane, 1997) lists 10 key design principles. The last principle is "adapt to disease continuum," meaning that the environment needs to be monitored and adapted to one's changing needs. To me, this is a perfect argument for creating a successful design for *nonsegregated* living.

While working at St. John's Home in Rochester, New York, I attended a design symposium in London in 2009 where the plans for our first community of Green House® homes were presented, along with many other designs. At one point during the symposium, the panel engaged in a lively discussion about appropriate design features for those living with dementia. In the midst of the debate, moderator David Hughes, an architect from the British firm Pozzoni, LLC, joined the discussion and declared, "Good design for dementia is good design for people!" Amen to that.

I had a chance to test that theory on a return engagement in England. Part of my involvement as a speaker at the 2012 U.K. Dementia Congress was an invitation to moderate a panel presentation of architectural designs for three housing complexes for people living with dementia. (In a wonderful irony, the conference organizers had forgotten about my stance on segregated living when they named me the moderator.) Each community was beautifully designed, and much was made of the special features that were incorporated.

I had no interest in dragging the architects into a full-scale debate about the segregation issue. But during the discussion, I mentioned Hughes's quote and expressed the opinion that many of their touted design features (such as hallways without dead ends, easy access to the outdoors, abundant natural light, and homey, farm-style kitchens) were features that I would also enjoy as a person without dementia. I asked each of the three panelists if there was anything about his or her design that specifically demanded a segregated living environment in order to work, or that only people with dementia might find beneficial and pleasing. All three said, "No, not really."

Community-Based Living and Identity

For people living in the community, it might seem at first glance that identity would be better preserved, as people living in their own homes continue to be surrounded by family members, personal possessions, and other trappings of their lives. To a certain extent, this is true; a person living at home does not need to deal with double rooms or a shared living space that is based on the presence of her dementia.

However, for those living with dementia, there is still much in their own home to challenge their identity. First, all of the stigmas of dementia already described in this chapter, from "zombies" to "fading away" to "dying twice," are lived out in the day-to-day interactions between a person living with dementia and her family, friends, and healthcare professionals in all settings. Second, the approach to care, even though it does not look institutional on the surface, nevertheless can create a similar degree of institutional living.

There is little financial support for home-based care, and many people living with dementia have a spouse (usually also an older adult) or a son or daughter (who often is also a working parent) providing the bulk of support. As a result, one's personal choices for awakening, bedtimes, meals, and personal care may succumb to the needs of the people trying to provide that support while going about their busy days. When contracted home services are used, they also often set their visits around the agency's needs, not those of each individual they serve.

If home-based care partners do not see the person as a whole individual and make an effort to learn her history, the same ingredients for misunderstanding a person's needs exist in her own home as in the nursing home. A lack of appreciation or compensation for one's unique rhythms or activity patterns often leads to sundown symptoms in the home. The inability of family members to flex their routines around one member's changing biorhythms also leads them to seek prescriptions for nighttime sedation, which can actually hasten her disengagement and decline.

If our own identity needs to be preserved by our social network, this broader support can be equally broken in the community, where people find themselves increasingly isolated after the diagnosis. As a result, the friends and family who represent all of the facets of our lives—our relationships, occupation, religious and leisure pursuits—slowly withdraw and with them goes a large part of the identity we are struggling so much to preserve:

> After I was diagnosed, my friends stopped coming around to see me. Finally, I called one of them and asked him, "Why don't you come to see me anymore?" He said, "Richard, I just didn't know what to say." I said to him, "How about 'Hello'?" (Taylor, 2011)

Finally, the societal stigma of dementia creates a loss of identity, not only for the person living with the illness, but for her loved ones as well. The word *stigma* means a mark given to criminals, slaves, or other undesirable people, indicating their status to others around them. In the case of the social stigma of dementia, the mark does not simply stick to the person with the diagnosis; it also leaps onto those who associate with her, most particularly her close family members. The result is isolation of family care partners as well, producing a further loss of identity. They are avoided, either because the reality of their loved one's illness is too difficult for people to confront, or because it is assumed that they are no longer available to engage in normal relations due to the situation they have inherited. The individuals slowly merge into a single nonperson, and they often either withdraw or are excluded from community life.

Many family members see placement in a nursing home as a sign of a failure on their part to provide the care a loved one needs. But it is not their fault. The system of support we have in the community is limited and, therefore, is not flexible enough to adapt to an individualized approach. In other words, the person's home has become an institution as well, and her identity is often lost among her very own family members and personal surroundings.

In fact, a move to a residential living environment does not necessarily spell failure, and can have many positive effects. There may be more opportunities for socialization, and the presence of an enlightened care staff can often provide greater flexibility to meet the changing needs of the person. This also enables family members to once more assume a primary relational role, providing emotional and spiritual support. These are roles that have often become lost when the family member has to provide daily hands-on care; with care professionals assuming these tasks, the family can once again become the social support network that can advocate for and support the person's well-being. And, as is the theme of this chapter, an essential function of close relatives is to help care professionals understand those aspects of identity that will help them to better know and support the person.

Enhancing Identity

Now that we have examined all of the ways in which identity can be lost, how might it be restored? Next, I will examine ways in which we can enhance identity, as well as the other six domains of well-being, via the three complementary pathways of personal, operational, and physical transformation mentioned in Chapter 2. Most of the chapters of this book also examine personal transformation from both intrapersonal and interpersonal aspects. Finally, I will address specific approaches that are particularly suited to either long-term care or community-living environments.

Personal Transformation

The first step in enhancing identity is to reject a narrow biomedical view of dementia and the stigma that results. The experiential definition is a good way to begin, for all the reasons detailed previously. Viewing a person living with dementia as a whole person whose experience of the world is shifting creates the mindset needed to move beyond our limitations and judgments.

The experiential model also tells us that the perspective of the person living with dementia is critical to our understanding of how best to support him. Anyone who engages in these efforts, from informal to professional care partners, will benefit from reading and listening to the words of those who are on this journey and seeking to understand their viewpoints, even if they do not match our own worldview.

From this comes the understanding that we cannot impose our own worldview on a person living with dementia any more than we can on our friends, relatives, or co-workers. Instead, we need to dig deeper into the person's history, collecting the stories that have defined him, and continue to support his ability to cope with the changes that he is experiencing.

When we learn to see each person as whole and unique, we temper the rules and generalizations we have been taught with the reality that each person expresses brain changes in his own way. We can then tailor this knowledge to better support individualized life and care.

Particularly in community-based living, one of the most important but confusing aspects of one's identity involves change. In other words, a person has a unique identity defined by his personal history, but he is also changing in a very individualized way as he lives with the symptoms of dementia. So we need to take what we know about our loved one and apply it to his life, but also be able to recognize when some aspects have changed irrevocably. This is not necessarily a bad thing; if part of a person's past identity can no longer be expressed in the present moment (or is no longer important to the person), it may need to be left behind to support the "new normal."

I often see family members struggle with this because they try to engage their loved one in "something he always loved to do," and when he is unable or shows disinterest, they assume he is incapable of any successful engagement. Or if he does not remember all that they are able to remember, they despair that he is no longer "with them." This describes the frustration that many people with dementia feel during reminiscence activities, or when they are quizzed by family members about names and faces of people from their past. Taylor (2011) feels that our stigmatized view of a person living with dementia leads us to test him repeatedly on past events and people, hoping he will answer enough of our questions correctly to prove to us that "Dad is still there."

> As a person with dementia, I am struggling to make sense of *today*; but as my caregivers, you only offer me *yesterday*.

These actions often arise from *our own* deep needs for reassurance and emotional stability, to protect ourselves from the burgeoning sense of loss that we face as care partners. But an experiential approach accepts that identity is more about who we are than what we can do, or what we can remember. Our memories and abilities may change as we age, but that should not define us.

An example I often give from my own life is that I used to run on the college cross-country team. I was not the star of the team, but at that time in my life I could run a lot farther and faster than most of my peers. I cannot run that far or that fast anymore, so my efforts to stay in shape have revolved around exercise goals that are more attainable for someone my age, rather than for a 21-year-old. My life is no less meaningful, and I focus on my strengths and try not to spend too much time grieving over that which I can no longer do. When it comes to sports, one could say that I also have a "new normal."

Fazio (2008) beautifully summarizes this tricky balance of past and present identity, which he describes as "the evolving self":

> It is important to connect with who the person is currently, to support who the person has been throughout his or her life, and to stay open to exploring who he or she is becoming. The past must be allowed to influence the present, yet not to define it. The present must also be allowed to influence the present. At the same time, both the past and present must be allowed to shape the future, and the future must be left free to influence itself. (p. 117)

Thus, supporting the evolving self is a dance that modifies its steps as the abilities and priorities of the person change over time. What is the correct mix of past and present? Whatever mix creates the greatest degree of well-being. If an aspect of the past clearly causes a person distress, it is a clue that the person is evolving beyond that part of his identity, and needs to find a new foothold that supports his present self *and* helps him succeed into the future.

An interesting extension of this concept is the way in which important facets of one's past identity can emerge as unmet needs when they can no longer be realized in the traditional manner. For example, a person who retains a strong identity as a parent and nurturer may search for her children or attempt to help those around her to walk, assist them with their meals, and so forth. Such expressions are often narrowly viewed as "delusions" or "challenging behaviors" when in fact they are a symbolic expression of a meaningful part of the person's identity that she cannot express in her present circumstance. As we will see, recognizing these aspects of identity are a crucial part of a new approach (discussed further in Chapters 7 and 10).

From an *interpersonal* standpoint, there is a variety of ways that we can enhance identity through our daily interactions. One of the most basic (and often neglected) ways is to ask how a person prefers to be addressed. All too often, whether in the nursing home or in the community, professional staff will automatically call a person by his first name, a familiarity that may not be appropriate to the relationship. In fact, using first names with older adults also perpetuates our view of such people as being dependent, or even child-like.

> The father of a close friend developed dementia due to a series of strokes, and eventually needed to move to a nursing home. He was a retired physician, an "old-school" doctor who also had provided support to his wife (who was legally blind), until he became unable to do so.
>
> After moving to the nursing home, my friend reported to me that her father had a number of altercations with the staff, often becoming angry and resisting their attempts to care for him. In our discussions, it was clear that much of this related to his loss of autonomy in the nursing home environment, especially given his long history as an authority figure and one who had cared for others.
>
> In exploring this further, I learned that the staff generally addressed him by his first name. This seemed inappropriate, given his previous identity. I suggested to my friend that she ask the staff to address him as "Dr. Hills," instead of "David." This simple recognition of his identity helped to improve his interactions with staff. I also believe it helped them to see him in a different light and treat him with more respect.

A deep knowledge of a person's past and present enables us to hone other communication skills as well. We can discover the best techniques for facilitating engagement and understanding by bringing in other aspects of identity (such as favorite music) to bridge broken pathways to understanding and even improve functional ability.

> Mark lives in one of St. John's Home's community Green House homes in Penfield, New York—two homes nestled within a multigenerational residential community that house 10 people each and provide skilled care (the first of its kind in the nation). A former football player and phys. ed. teacher, Mark has a dementia that is felt to be due to chronic traumatic encephalopathy.
>
> Part of Mark's difficulty lies in his ability to process and follow commands. He seems to understand many instructions, but cannot translate them to the physical act that is described. Often his feet get "stuck," and it is hard for him to walk, even with verbal cuing.
>
> However, music unlocks Mark's legs. He dances quite nimbly when music is played. His care partners have learned that the use of music often helps him to overcome his walking difficulties, and that singing to him helps him lift his feet and move along.

Another example of enhancing identity through music can be seen with Dan Cohen's "Music and Memory" project (www.musicandmemory.org). The use of portable music players with personalized music can have dramatic effects on the abilities of people with dementia, reawakening memories and facilitating engagement. This project was profiled in the film *Alive Inside* (Ximotion Media, 2013), which received the Audience Award for Best U.S. Documentary at the 2014 Sundance Film Festival. The film features several people who had been disengaged and unable to communicate clearly or recognize family members. After spending time listening to music that is chosen to tie into his or her past, each person becomes more engaged, speaks more fluently, and retrieves memories more effectively. Some sing or get up and dance, astounding their care partners. Another surprising finding is that these abilities persist for several hours after the music stops and the headphones are removed, suggesting that many cognitive abilities are not completely destroyed, but simply require a novel "key" to unlock them.

The key to Cohen's success is the use of *personalized* music. This approach uses identity to optimize the results of the music in a way that a generic music program cannot. The domain of identity can enrich the use of music, art, and many other forms of engagement.

There are many more ways that care partners can shift their interpersonal approaches than can be mentioned here. Once again, maximizing our understanding of the person's unique, if evolving, identity is what counts. And as we partner with people to support their evolving self, our own self evolves to become more empathic, intuitive, and skilled in this "dance":

> In the dance between these worlds, the person with forgetfulness leads and you, the helper, follow. One step forward, two steps backwards; one moment more over here, another moment over there. You are a messenger between worlds. (Shabahangi & Szymkiewicz, 2008, p. 42)

In her early days of public speaking about caring for her husband, Joseph, who lived with Alzheimer's, Sarah Rowan used to bring Joseph with her when he was able. One day, she experienced this dance quite literally:

> I often think of living with dementia as the "delicate dance." Once when I was speaking about Alzheimer's disease, Joseph, who had accompanied me, arose, took my hand, and began to dance with me. So while I spoke about our experience, we continued to dance together in front of the crowd. I saw this as a transitional moment. . . . With every step, Joseph was teaching me how to move from the life we had known together to a new shared existence. Sometimes, it's a tango; another time, it may be a waltz. You never know. . . . All I had to do was stay open . . . and follow. . . . (Brilliant Image Productions, 2012)

Operational Transformation

In long-term care settings, there are many operational changes that can help enhance identity. As we will see with each well-being domain, these involve both the creation of new operational processes and the reversal of old ones that have been working against one's well-being.

A central operational process that has been stuck in the narrow biomedical approach is the process of welcoming people to the home and planning their care. This begins with an "admission," in which the newly arrived person (often weak from a recent hospitalization and/or traumatized by the move) is put through a series of interviews and assessments that are mostly centered on her medical conditions and cognitive and functional deficits.

Once again, the information that is obtained in these assessments is important and needs to be understood by the people working in the home. The process, however, has several limitations. Due to entrenched dysfunctions in our systems for transferring information between care environments, information that was previously known is usually solicited anew, in case the records were incorrect or incomplete. Even within the nursing home, the doctor, nurse, social worker, and various therapists often ask many of the same questions. This can be physically and emotionally exhausting for the person, which in turn may affect her cognitive and physical performance on those assessments.

Another limitation of this process is that its strong biomedical focus starts everyone off on the track of not seeing the whole person. And the excess disability that results from this exhausting gauntlet of assessments leads us to underestimate a person's capabilities, and it creates a strong foundation for a paternalistic approach to care. The collection of any personal information often falls upon the social worker or activity professional to solicit, and even those reports are often lacking, particularly if the person is forgetful or if fatigue or delirium persist due to a recent illness.

Embedded within this process is the "admission care plan," which is prepared several days to weeks after the person moves in. While generally touted as an opportunity to hear more about the person from himself and his family, the care plan too often follows the same pattern of outlining all of one's various medical illnesses and deficits, and the staff's plan to address these. It is commonly charted as an abbreviated list of deficits—"alteration in blood sugar," "alteration in cognitive status," and so forth—with a biomedically focused solution for each. The whole person is thereby reduced to a series of diseases and tasks.

A more holistic assessment seeks to learn about such factors as one's core identity, leisure enjoyment, spirituality, personality strengths and challenges, communication styles, responses to stressors, or unique talents and abilities. In speaking about this process, I often remind audiences that I am much more than the sum of my medical conditions, and I am also much more than a list of the things I do not do particularly well. Any doctor, nurse, or therapist who tries to address my needs without understanding who I am, what I value, and what I continue to do well fails to meet the standards of good practice.

The first step for transforming organizations is to recognize the drawbacks of the existing model, and to enlist a working group to re-imagine the process of welcoming someone to the home. This working group should represent a variety of disciplines, and ideally one or more elders and family members as well. Professionals need to gain an understanding of how people experience the traditional admission process. Stories of individual experiences should be solicited from those who have recently arrived as well as from their family members.

It is also beneficial to role-play the process; some homes have placed staff members on a gurney at the front door, wheeled them through the building to the living area, and transferred them onto a bed in one of the rooms. Participants are often shocked at the feelings they experience—the embarrassment of being transported past a multitude of people in this manner, the inability to see anything but the ceiling tiles going by, or the impersonal reception they often experience upon their arrival.

Culture change consultants Barbara Frank and Cathie Brady often take workshop participants through a visualization of this process. Participants are asked to think about what they would need most when they first arrive in their room after transfer from a hospital. Their personal wishes—a warm smile and greeting, a trip to the bathroom, a pain medication after the trip, a kind touch, or simply a bit of quiet solitude to recover from the move—are often not practiced in the participants' homes.

Armed with this knowledge, the working group can then create a moving-in process that better recognizes identity. They can identify what clinical data must be confirmed and how best to do so without redundancy and exhaustion. They can challenge the need to have all data collected on day one, creating space for physical and psychological recovery, and thus promoting comfort and familiarity with the new environment.

To advocate for slowing down the intensity of the assessment process while broadening our knowledge of the whole person may seem like a contradiction. However, by role-playing this process and incorporating feedback from elders and families, the organization can create a more organic process whereby the newly arrived person can gradually become familiar with, and familiar to, his care partners, thereby creating a more durable and holistic identity that improves his well-being and clinical care.

> While speaking at an organizational retreat in Edmonton, Alberta, for the Good Samaritan Society homes, I learned of a nice process one of the homes had adopted to help make the initial care plan more holistic. They recognized that there was often a large amount of clinical material that had to be addressed at the meeting, which invariably shoved the rest of the person's identity to the side.
>
> Their solution was to change the mindset of the people who were attending the meeting *before* the fact. They did this by holding a brief "get-to-know-you" meeting within a few days of the arrival of the elder and his or her family members, in which the various workers could learn about the person outside of the illness.
>
> What they have found is that even though the subsequent care plan might have a great deal of clinical information to impart, the staff members arrived at the meeting seeing a much broader identity for the person in question, and the discussion was much more holistic and strength-based as a result.

It may seem like such a process of building identity is too complex to be practically applied in a long-term care setting. But there is evidence it can succeed, because many organizations are transitioning to very similar processes to improve identity among new employees. St. John's Home in Rochester, New York, along with many other homes, has moved beyond the traditional interview/hiring/orientation paradigm to create a more organic process of assimilation into the organization over the first 6 months to a year, one that recognizes a person's need to build familiarity and capabilities over time.

And just as a new employee would be expected to develop and hone skills over time, this new view helps us see the potential of the person with dementia to actually improve in several cognitive and functional domains as he acclimates to his environment. One even wonders whether an overreliance on assessments performed immediately upon arrival forces us to see the person as being less capable, thereby creating a care plan that does not enable such improvement to occur. We will discuss this and other "self-fulfilling prophecies" in the chapters to come.

Another barrier to making a more gradual transition in U.S. nursing homes is the posthospital reimbursement system, which drives rapid assessment and institution of rehabilitative therapies and cuts off such funding as soon as the person fails to make significant functional gains. The irony is that if the person were given a week's rest after moving to the home, he might actually perform better in therapy and reach a higher level of ability, but our system rarely gives the home a chance to find out.

Once a new process of moving in has been realized, the care plan itself is the next item to be tackled. Because most people conflate care with medical treatment, organizations need to use these concepts of well-being to demonstrate that a plan that focuses simply on medical and nursing treatments is too narrow to serve the whole person. Instead, many organizations have switched to "wellness plans," "growth plans," or "life plans," and have constructed documents that preserve the medical information, but embed it into a more comprehensive view of the person and his goals.

Another way to help preserve identity is to write such plans in narrative form, expressed in the first person (even if the person is not able to speak to you). This brings not only a sense of identity into the document, but also a sense of agency, or person-direction. Many homes have moved down this path, and organizations such as The Eden Alternative® (www.edenalt.org) and the Pioneer Network (www.pioneer network.net) have resources to help homes get started.

The Colorado-based technology company It's Never 2 Late (www. IN2L.com) helps organizations create video care plans with personalized images that further strengthen identity. Life histories are another important resource, and organizations such as Ohio-based LifeBio (www.lifebio.com) have tools to help people in all living environments create a life history with and for their care partners. The best such documents are more than a laundry list of "facts" about the person's past—instead, they are a chronicle of the people and experiences that have shaped the person throughout her life, as well as her reflections on life, capturing her wisdom and unique perspective and creating a legacy for future generations.

Dedicated Staff Assignments

If knowing a person's identity is a key to providing good care, it follows that the best care arises from close and continuous contact. Bell and Troxel (1997) express this concept as the Best Friends™ approach, founded on the principle that we best support people living with dementia through the same set of values we would follow with our closest friends. Needless to say, one cannot be a "best friend" to someone with whom you only interact sporadically.

This leads to the topic of dedicated staff assignments, whether in home-based care or in the nursing home. This seems to be a very difficult practice for most organizations to embrace, and yet it is one of the most critical components of high-quality care for people living with dementia. There are two benefits to this operational approach: the professional care partners become more familiar with the person, and thus are better able to understand her needs, and the person who is forgetful has a better chance of forming durable memories of those who provide her care, thus building a level of comfort and trust. As we will see, this also feeds into other well-being domains, particularly connectedness and security. (Chapter 4 includes a very thorough discussion of dedicated staff assignments.)

The Power of Language

A final operational aspect that deserves mention is intentional use of language that will enhance identity, not destroy it. By understanding the ways in which we create stigma and reinforce limited views of a person, we can choose language that moves us to a new level of thinking. Here are a few examples:

- The word *patient* puts the person squarely in the arena of disease and medical treatment. We are all patients at one time or another, but we are always people first, and our word choices should reflect that. Therefore, a "dementia patient" can be better described as a "person living with (the symptoms of) dementia."

- The phrase *living with* is also a better alternative to *suffering from* or *victim of*, as it reminds us that there are continued opportunities for well-being, whereas the other terms are fatalistic and suggest that suffering is the only path available.

- Many phrases used to describe what we observe in people are judgmental and pejorative, from *behavior problems* to *being difficult, being bad, acting out*, or even *wandering* (which suggests purposeless rather than need-directed activity).

- Many terms, such as *paranoid* or *delusional*, are improperly applied and often ascribe psychiatric illness to expressions that may be entirely justifiable from the perspective of a person living with dementia. This can lead to misuse of psychotropic medication.

There are many more terms and phrases that can destroy identity. The Pioneer Network website has an extensive list, along with suggested alternatives. They also invite users of the site to submit terms of their own that they feel need to be updated. Many more terms were identified in *Dementia Beyond Drugs*. I have chosen not to rehash them here, but rather to move forward with intentional use of language that enhances well-being.

Physical Transformation

A physical environment that best supports identity is one that is personalized and optimizes familiarity. There are many resources that describe ways to personalize living spaces in long-term care, so this discussion will be limited to a few aspects that are often underappreciated.

It is common to use items from a person's past to decorate her living area. This reflects our knowledge that long-term memory tends to be better preserved than recent memory. It may help preserve identity, but it also reflects our own tendency to focus on the person's memory. When looking at the evolving self, we need to periodically audit the environment to determine if this approach is truly benefiting the person.

Some people become confused by objects that are presented out of time, such as when they are shown photos of relatives long deceased, or when family portraits show their children at a much younger age than they are today. Familiarity, therefore, needs to be created by using objects that we recognize, but that do not create too much disconnect from our understanding of our present situation. A person's tendency to become "unstuck in time" will vary through her life with dementia, and understanding how she is currently experiencing the flow of time will help guide care partners with regard to the mix of past and present that should make up her living space.

Additionally, personalization is about more than adding objects; it can also be about feeling a sense of familiarity and control (reflecting the domains of security and autonomy). Therefore, having the person rearrange the space and helping to create a place that feels safe, familiar, and comforting are also very important, even when the person is only residing there for the short term. This will be addressed further in Chapters 5 and 6.

Another way to increase familiarity and minimize confusion is to *engage* the person in conversation about her physical environment. This is more than simple reminiscence over photos. It is an examination of various objects in the person's living space, along with a gently guided conversation about her connection to them and what they represent in the context of her life, past and present. This gives a forgetful person the degree of repetition needed to keep memories durable, and it also helps care partners to see if the object is still of value in supporting her evolving self, or if it may be counterproductive.

In congregate living environments, there is often little personalization outside of one's bedroom or apartment. Therefore, it is also important to engage the person in exploring the shared spaces, with an emphasis on reinforcing familiar aspects throughout, such as a favorite chair in the lounge, an aquarium, a household pet, or a favorite view from a window. Personal artwork can also be used to decorate common areas, instead of stock art from the local department store.

Once again, knowledge of the person's identity helps us create familiarity through those aspects of shared spaces that are most meaningful to the person. An avid gardener might be regularly engaged with the home's gardens and indoor plants, a meteorologist might be engaged in watching the weather outside, and someone who loved to cook might be engaged in watching or participating in the preparation of food in an accessible kitchen.

When we look past the pure "trappings" of one's former home, and instead focus on creating meaningful interactions with the current physical environment, we realize another benefit that often goes unrecognized in long-term care: The person is able to form new memories, and her identity evolves to encompass, even embrace, the new living space, including new activities and experiences. Too much preoccupation with preserving the past may actually delay her ability to acclimate and make sense of the new environment. While the building may be unfamiliar, it is the tie-in to identity (and to the other domains to follow) more than the physical trappings that will determine when and if a person will adjust and feel comfortable in her new living space.

One final note: Understanding the physical attributes of the living environment that trigger identity can also give clues to the meaning behind certain actions:

> During a speaking trip to Iowa in 2011, I heard the story of a gentleman who lived in an assisted living home in a rural part of the state. He was repeatedly attempting to exit the back door, and each time was redirected by his care partners, who did not feel he was safe walking outside alone. His attempts to go outside became more insistent with each redirection.

Finally, the administrator suggested that the staff not interfere the next time he opened the door, but simply watch from the doorway, to see what he might be trying to accomplish. When they did so, the gentleman walked to the fence at the back of the yard, which adjoined a cow pasture. He watched the cattle grazing for about 10 minutes, and then turned around and came back inside.

In soliciting more information about the gentleman, they learned from his family that he had been a farmer who would go out every day to "check on the cows." This pattern was being repeated at the home, and once this longstanding practice was revealed, he was able to do so daily, with the knowledge that his identity was being preserved and his need fulfilled.

This is a good example of why our attempts at nonpharmacological interventions, and our research studies of these interventions, often produce disappointing results. We may try aromatherapy, music, or laundry folding, when maybe the person simply needs to "check on the cows"! Now that we have rediscovered the *person*, let us reconnect him with the world.

CHAPTER 4

Connectedness

I once thought a person could live alone and devote a life to the mind. I outlined a play with such a theme. The main character was a man on display at a zoo. It has taken thirty years for me to realize why I couldn't finish the play.

—Thomas DeBaggio

No man is an island,
Entire of itself.
Each is a piece of the continent,
A part of the main . . .

—John Donne

Connectedness Defined

FOX ET AL. (2005) DEFINE the well-being domain of *connectedness* as a "state of being connected; alive; belonging; engaged; involved; not detached; connected to the past, present, and future; connected to personal possessions; connected to place; connected to nature." I would add that these connections also go beyond the tangible to include spirituality, creativity, love, and hope.

For most of us, our lives are largely spent seeking connections—with family, friends, and people who share geography, occupations, avocations, culture, or faith traditions. Even those who spend large parts of their lives seeking solitude are also seeking connections of the intangible or nonhuman kind. Given the crisis in identity brought on by the experience of dementia, it is not surprising that connections of all sorts are seriously challenged, often from the day the diagnosis is spoken out loud.

We will explore these challenges further in this chapter, but before we delve into them, a word of caution: Each of the seven domains of well-being exists in resonance with the person's network of support, whether familial, professional, or social. When we follow practices that erode well-being for the individual, we may ultimately erode our own as well.

A major drawback of the biomedical view of dementia is the way in which it produces stigmatized views (such as those described in Chapter 3) that create separation between so-called normal individuals and the person living with a cognitive disability. Sabat, Johnson, Swarbrick, and Keady (2011) refer to this stigmatized image as "the demented other," and argue that the use of such labeling language only "reinforces [the] divide" (p. 282).

A major advantage of the experiential model is that it highlights the *commonalities* between the two groups by describing the process of cognitive change in terms that are nonjudgmental of the person with dementia and also could be applied in various degrees to all of us, as our life experiences bring about an evolution of our own perspective on the world.

If we succumb to a view that creates an "us" and "them" mentality, we become blind to better ways of caring and support; we also create a system by which each of us could become disenfranchised, should our views or abilities deviate from the accepted practices of mainstream society. Keeping people who live with dementia connected ultimately assures a better future for each of us, and the converse is also true. After all, the poem by Donne concludes with this admonition:

> Therefore, send not to know
> For whom the bell tolls,
> It tolls for thee.

How Dementia Challenges Connectedness

For the domain of connectedness, we will look at intrinsic challenges from a microscopic perspective, and then zoom outward when looking at extrinsic challenges.

Intrinsic Challenges

The biological process of cognitive illness results from a multitude of disrupted connections. The end point of damage in all such illnesses is the nerve cells and the connections (structural and functional) that they form with one another. So, at its most basic level, dementia is about broken connections. These include connections with how our thoughts and sensory input are processed, how we are able to respond to our environment and communicate needs, and how we access memory and a variety of cognitive skills, from wayfinding to problem solving.

The person living with dementia feels these challenges to connectedness very early on, even before he may be ready to accept the reality of his illness. He can quickly become frustrated by loved ones who "don't seem to listen to me" or "forgot what I just told them," and often the ability to find the words to express himself is affected early, as in Ed Voris's story (see Chapter 1).

First-person narratives are rich with descriptions of these feelings of separation and alienation:

> When you feel like a whole person, you are in control of yourself and of your surroundings. I don't have that feeling of control any longer. Is it forgotten? If there is a spark of that feeling left, it is almost unreachable for me. It is like having your head in a fish bowl. You can see out, but nothing can get in. (Rose, 2003, p. 1)

> Yet half my life seems to be spent searching for things. I don't want to say that objects I am trying to find have been lost or misplaced. I simply can't remember where any transient object might be. As soon as I put down a hat or a shirt in an unusual place, it becomes "lost." Half my life now seems to be spent looking for things. It often seems that Alzheimer's is making all kinds of things disappear. (DeBaggio, 2002, p. 124)

One principle that will repeat itself throughout these pages is that the seven domains of well-being are not mutually exclusive—they feed into one another in multiple ways. Erosion of one domain can affect the next; fortunately, the inverse is also true when well-being domains are enhanced. In the case of connectedness, we see a particularly close tie to identity; it is hard to discuss one without the other coming into play. The preceding quotes reflect this as well.

With loss of memory, the world around you becomes one of disconnectedness, as objects from both past and present may lose their meaning, or you may lose the narrative that gives them meaning for you. Cognitive changes can also create difficulties in filtering out competing stimuli, such that background noise can make it harder for a person to focus on a conversation or activity, which can lead to withdrawal.

We could produce many more examples of broken connections, but the experiential view teaches us to look at these intrinsic changes from more than a deficit-based view. So instead of expanding further upon purely negative experiences, let us explore some other intrinsic aspects of one's changing connectedness that are less easily recognized and may hold keys to strength-based approaches.

Humans (and human brains) are endlessly adaptable to changes and challenges. The brain of a person living with dementia is no exception. A more holistic view reminds us that, even in people who live with severe cognitive disability, there are millions of neurons working perfectly well. And their brains continue to work to compensate for the broken connections, just as a person with a stroke learns to compensate for a paralyzed limb. Even a heavily affected brain continues to adjust to adversity—problem solving, creating new maps and new narratives, or calling on novel nerve pathways to process and respond to information presented to it. In other words, *what is commonly seen as confused or challenging behavior is, in actuality, compensatory or adaptive behavior by an individual who continues to express agency and purpose in his own unique way.*

Another example of the adapting brain is the heightened sensitivity many people have to nonverbal communication and subtle attributes of the environment that may go unnoticed by others. Such sensitivity is likely due to an unmasking or a growth of this level of perception, when areas of the brain concerned with memory and verbal skills become affected. A loss in one area leads to compensation in another.

Sturm et al. (2013) look at this phenomenon and propose a mechanism for the structural changes in the temporal lobe that unmask this ability. Unfortunately, while their theory has merit, they continue to view the process strictly from a deficit-based perspective; they refer to this heightened environmental sensitivity as "emotional contagion," likening it to an infectious disease.

Do we need to see this merely as a sign of pathology? After all, we do not usually view the exquisite hearing of blind people as a disease process, even though it is a similar form of compensation. While such heightened sensitivity can often be a trigger for distress, it could also be seen as a gift. We can learn a great deal about nonverbal communication and the subtle effects of the living environment from people living with dementia. (I share several examples of this in Chapters 5, 7, and 8.)

A second concept in reframing our view of broken connections is that shifting abilities will necessarily shift one's priorities. As with my personal example in the last chapter, my changing ability to compete at sports has led me to prioritize how much time and effort I devote to that part of my life, relative to other skills and experiences. Similarly, a person whose cognitive functions are challenged may find it best to "let go" of certain ways of connecting that are too difficult to maintain, in favor of others. When the person does not prioritize the way we think he should, we see him as confused or challenging, but too often we are forcing our own judgment on him, rather than understanding what works best in his current situation.

Examples of this concept in relation to connectedness include (1) people declining certain programmed activities over the objections of care partners who feel it is in their best interest to force such engagement; (2) family members correcting a person who misstates names, or who does not remember an event exactly the way they do; or (3) the all-too-common debate over the value of "reorientation therapy," particularly as a response to a statement that we consider to be confused.

This leads to a third, very important concept: As a result of their need to compensate for broken connections, people living with dementia view the world through a very different lens than we do. Our lack of appreciation of this causes us to repeatedly misidentify needs and respond inadequately to those needs. Once again, the clue to this breakthrough in communication and support comes from one of our True Experts, Christine Bryden.

In *Dementia Beyond Drugs*, I closed the book with a quote from Bryden (2005) that includes the observation that people with dementia are making "an important journey from cognition, through emotion, into spirit" (p. 159). This somewhat unassuming statement contains one of the most powerful lessons care partners can learn when it comes to connectedness.

To me, what Bryden's statement says is that many people who lose a strong connection with a world dominated by memories, facts, and logic reorganize their thoughts and express themselves from a perspective dominated by emotions, feelings, and symbolism. The challenge to connectedness is that we often do not realize this and continue to try to answer their needs from our perspective, using facts and logic to try to "bring them into our world," which amounts to a failed tactic. I will explain how this knowledge opens up a new approach later in the chapter, when I discuss ways to enhance connectedness.

Extrinsic Challenges

With the close tie between identity and connectedness, it is clear that many of the extrinsic challenges to connectedness result from the narrow biomedical view of the person with dementia and the stigmas it creates. Chapter 3 described how a view of a person as "half empty" or "fading away" could isolate both the person and her family members from others. If personhood is partly dependent on relationships within a social context, this relationship can be quickly lost if the person is seen as "no longer there."

When a person's ability to relate to others is challenged by difficulties with memory and communication skills, it requires additional skill on the part of the care partner to enable effective communication. If such skills are lacking, or if it is assumed that the person can no longer communicate due to her illness, then connections are broken and our low expectations create another cycle of self-fulfilling prophecy.

The first time I met Dr. Richard Taylor in 2009, we were both speaking at Alzheimer's Disease International in Singapore. I introduced myself shortly after Richard's keynote, and reflected on a comment he had made about how he is seen by others. He responded that as soon as people hear that he has Alzheimer's, he can detect a shift in their facial expressions, tone of voice, and the way in which they speak to him, even though the conversation had been perfectly unremarkable up to that point. Such is the extent to which the societal view of dementia has affected our subconscious minds.

In his own account of living with Alzheimer's, Reverend Robert Davis (1989) echoes this experience:

> As soon as I was diagnosed, some people became very uncomfortable around me. I realize that the shock and pain, especially to those who have a parent with the disease, are difficult to deal with at first. It was strange that in most cases I had to make the effort to seek out people who were avoiding me and look them in the eye and say, "I don't bite. I am still the same person. I just can't do my work anymore. . . . I am still at home in here, and I need your friendship and acceptance."
>
> Usually the response was one of great relief. Over and over the answer came, "I'm so glad you said that. I just didn't know what to

say. I didn't know how to treat you. I didn't know if you could still laugh." (p. 100)

Cary Smith Henderson (1998) expresses similar frustrations with social engagement:

> And another really crazy thing about Alzheimer's, nobody really wants to talk to you any longer. They're maybe afraid of us, I don't know if that's the trouble or not, I assume it is, but we can assure everybody that we know Alzheimer's is not catching. (p. 18)

When people converse with a married couple, this bias expresses itself in a tendency to speak primarily to the unaffected spouse, even if the statement would be more appropriately directed to the person living with dementia. Many people have told me that this is particularly infuriating when it occurs in conversations with their physicians.

Much of this type of stigma reaches well beyond cognitive illnesses. Older people in general may be overlooked in conversations and, sadly, it is all too common in long-term care to have care partners and family members discuss a person as if she is not in the room. This phenomenon is also commonly seen as gender bias in younger adults, such as a mechanic or repairman speaking to the husband, even if his wife is asking the questions. Thus, it should be very easy for us to appreciate the frustration that such exclusion might cause.

Robert Simpson (Simpson & Simpson, 1999) describes the interplay that occurred between stigma and connectedness when he and his wife were engaged in conversations with others:

> People instinctively talk to you. It's like I'm nothing. Oh, they'll say, "Hi, Bob," but right away they start visiting with *you*, and I'll just stand there. It used to be that they would talk to me, too. But I was more sure of myself then, I could take a more aggressive stance and start a conversation. Now I know I make people anxious. I'm sure I pick up more vibrations now. . . . I don't seem all that different to myself, but people treat me differently when they know I have Alzheimer's. (p. 39)

Later in the book, Bob and his wife, Ann, have a further dialogue about how they struggle with connectedness with each other as well. Ann describes how her anticipatory grief creates a barrier, and Bob responds by reminding her that the traditional caregiver focus on *doing* often blinds us to other ways that connections can be maintained:

(Ann): Perhaps I do run around the edges of my pain to avoid the center of it. Maybe I do pull away from Bob. I take over his tasks, projecting ahead—always ahead—to the time when Bob will not be here and, in the process, I shut him out.

(Bob): I know you're busy now. You have so much to do. And I can't even help you! Do you remember when we first met—how we would just *be* together? We'd talk and laugh and not really do anything. (p. 99)

In skilled care settings, all of the foregoing intrinsic and extrinsic challenges apply; but connectedness is particularly challenged by physical and operational factors as well. The most basic physical challenge to connectedness is the very move to long-term care, away from family, home, neighbors, faith communities, cherished outdoor space—all that surrounded the person before the move.

In addition to the separation from home, the physical layout of the typical nursing home or assisted living home is on a larger scale, which creates greater distance between one's bedroom and the other places where life's daily activities may occur. It may be a long walk to a dining room or living room, and access to the outdoors may be all but impossible in multistory buildings where people are not able to move about independently.

The Critical Importance of Dedicated Staffing Patterns

The biggest operational barrier to connectedness arises from the tendency of most homes to rotate staff, such that a person sees a parade of different faces providing care and support from month to month. This seems to suit the staffing needs of many organizations when viewed purely through their lens, but the effect is devastating on people who are forgetful and need to build familiarity and trust with those who provide hands-on support.

It is amazing to me how underappreciated the negative effect of rotating staff can be among nursing home leaders and hands-on care partners alike. I often lead people through a series of questions to try to drive the point home:

How many of you would like to see a different doctor every time you have an appointment? How about a different hairdresser? A different lawyer? If they all have access to your information, does that mean that you will be equally satisfied with any substitutes?

> Now, think about how it would feel to have one of your co-
> workers strip you naked and bathe you, or help you on and off
> the toilet. Is anyone here willing to pick a co-worker and give it
> a try? If that seems too difficult for you to imagine, think about
> having a different co-worker bathe you every few weeks. How
> much worse would this be for your own comfort and dignity?
> How can we ask people who are forgetful and feeling vulnerable
> to experience this indignity day after day, just to simplify our
> own routines?

My colleague, Dr. Emi Kiyota, lived in a nursing home for 3 weeks to experience such a life firsthand. She put one arm in a sling to mimic paralysis, confined herself to a wheelchair or armchair during the day, and asked the staff to care for her as they would any other resident of the home. Her baths consisted of bed-baths. These are described in the *Bathing without a Battle* video (Barrick, Rader, Hoeffer, Sloane, & Biddle, 2001), and are considered a very gentle and humane approach to bathing for those who find the traditional bath or shower to be too difficult. However, in Kiyota's case, a new staff member provided each successive bath. She also noted very little engagement or gentleness in the approach. She reports that, "By the time the third stranger in a row came in to remove my clothes and bathe me, I thought to myself, 'I have no dignity left'" (Kiyota, 2011).

As with my argument for integrated living environments, I could devote a section of each chapter to explain how dedicated staffing patterns enhance each domain of well-being. In the previous chapter, I discussed the importance of close relationships to enhance and maintain *identity*. To avoid too much repetition, I will address the importance of dedicated staffing for all of the remaining six domains of well-being here.

Connectedness is the perfect place to begin when stressing the importance of staffing patterns that nurture close and continuous relationships. Dedicated staffing fosters a sense of belonging for a person who is forgetful and may feel out of place in a nursing home environment. It also helps preserve a consistent and strong care-partner network for those who are still living in the community and have in-home services.

Looking at the other five domains, the advantages of dedicated staffing almost seem too obvious to list; and yet so many, if not most, organizations find this concept difficult to embrace.

To a great extent, a sense of *security* arises from familiarity. A familiar face or voice can do a lot to ease one's anxiety, whereas an unfamiliar face can easily have the opposite effect. These positive or negative effects are multiplied during those times when one's sense of security is most likely to be threatened, such as bathing, visiting a new environment, or attending a new activity.

Maximizing *autonomy* requires that we navigate the terrain of negotiated risk, a concept we will discuss in detail in Chapter 6. This cannot be safely accomplished without knowing the person and her values. When staffing assignments are rotated and people are less well known, the organization defaults to a broad-spectrum set of policies that place safety over quality of life and are inflexible to the needs of the individual.

Meaning ties into personal history, values, strengths, and passions. What is meaningful for one individual is not necessarily so for another. Creating meaningful experiences throughout the day requires a deeper understanding of a person than a casual acquaintance can provide. Once again, the common path for organizations that do not use dedicated staffing too often falls upon generic programming that meets their needs for documentation, but strips daily life of meaning for the individual. And in between programmed activities, such homes offer very little in the form of meaningful engagement, because staff members do not know the person well enough to create meaning in the moment.

Growth requires an environment that nurtures security, autonomy, and meaning. How does a stranger promote or measure personal growth in an individual who may not *do* very much by traditional functional scales?

Joy grows from the other six domains and is a much richer experience with friends than with strangers. Dedicated staffing also increases opportunities for spontaneity and the little personal touches that can enliven one's day and create joy.

Another overlooked advantage of dedicated staffing is that provided to the staff themselves. Rotating assignments between different living areas creates a repetitive process of forming and breaking work alliances that disrupts communication and collaboration. There is less investment in one's co-workers and a lesser tendency to hold to high standards of accountability.

Even when care partners are rotated within one living area, the constant shuffling of work assignments creates barriers to collaboration and flexibility, as each new rotation brings the need to re-learn patterns of interaction. Furthermore, the erosion of well-being for the elders served adds to the burden of conflict and frustration that arises from daily care. Dedicated assignments are, therefore, more efficient as well as more humane.

Many care partners express the need to have a break from elders or family members who are viewed as "challenging." However, much of the challenge arises from the frustration of those who feel that no one takes the time to understand them. Most organizations that move to dedicated assignments find that the level of conflict with elders and families decreases, because they are seen to be "in it for the long haul," rather than simply passing the buck when the going gets tough.

Beyond the advantages for well-being, dedicated staffing improves clinical care as well. The ability to identify and treat medical illness often hinges on recognizing subtle signs of change at a time when early intervention provides the greatest benefit. The earliest onset of an infection or other medical complication is often detected by a care partner (nurse or otherwise) whose familiarity with the person from day to day enables her to quickly detect that something has changed. I have received many timely calls because the dedicated care partner felt that someone "is not herself today." People who do not have deep familiarity with someone's baseline appearance often miss these cues.

Castle and Anderson (2011) surveyed 2,839 nursing homes in the United States, looking at four care outcomes (physical restraint use, urinary catheter use, pain management, and pressure ulcers). They found a significant improvement in care outcomes in homes that used dedicated staff assignments at a level of 80% or more.

Two further studies by Castle (2011) of 3,941 U.S. nursing homes showed that the number of survey-deficiency citations in several categories of quality of life and quality of care was significantly lower in homes with the highest level (85% or more) of dedicated nursing assistant staffing. Those homes also had significantly lower rates of turnover and absenteeism for nursing assistants (Castle, 2013).

Spector, Limcango, Williams, Rhodes, & Hurd (2013) found that as many as 60% of U.S. nursing home hospitalizations are potentially avoidable. The most common avoidable conditions included infections (especially urinary infections and pneumonia), congestive heart failure, delirium, dehydration, and falls. Each of these is a condition or event that can be better prevented when the person is well known and subtle changes are recognized. Furthermore, the study found that the presence of cognitive illness was a major risk factor for preventable hospitalizations; when a person's ability to communicate is impaired, the ability to "look past the words" and understand an individual becomes paramount.

The U.S. Centers for Medicare and Medicaid Services is considering new financial formulae that would pay an incentive to homes with low hospitalization rates, and/or penalize those with high rates. Therefore, using dedicated staffing to improve prevention and early detection is not only clinically superior, but will also produce better financial outcomes.

Kunik et al. (2010) and Morgan et al. (2013) looked at factors causing "aggressive behavior" in people living with dementia. Among the main causes found in each study was a decrease in the consistency and quality of contact between those people and their care partners.

All of the preceding points apply equally to those who provide in-home care services, services at day centers, or acute care hospitals, and for exactly the same reasons.

To summarize, dedicated assignments enhance well-being on multiple fronts, foster collaborative and accountable work environments, improve clinical care, reduce conflict, and improve satisfaction for people living with dementia and their families. Any organization that does not provide dedicated assignments offers a lower quality of care than they could otherwise. End of discussion.

Many culture change websites provide a list of suggested questions for prospective residents and their families to ask when touring elder care environments. Dedicated staffing is consistently included in these lists, and organizations can expect to be asked about this with increasing regularity.

Segregated Living and Connectedness

Depending on the organization's operational structure, there can be a variety of challenges to connectedness associated with segregated living environments. An initial move to "memory care" when a person displays forgetfulness prioritizes the illness over the important relationships developed with the people living and working in the person's previous environment, as well as the person's own familiarity with the environment.

Furthermore, many organizations group people in a stage-specific manner (which is a problem in itself, as no two people are alike, even if they display similar degrees of cognitive ability). Such organizations will tend to move people as their abilities change and they no longer "fit the program" for the unit, thus disrupting important connections, often repeatedly. Also, as seen with integrated environments, if care partners are rotated or outside contracted workers are brought in, the ability of the person to form knowing and trusting relationships is further compromised.

Because initiation of relationships is challenged by dementia, the ability to form and maintain such relationships is limited in segregated environments. While friendships undoubtedly occur between people living with dementia, the incorporation of people with normal cognition provides a different level of stimulation that can help keep people connected in a more durable way, which in turn can promote growth and maintenance of abilities. Integration also provides a care partnership role for the cognitively well person that can be highly fulfilling.

Community-Based Living and Connectedness

Most of the points discussed in the preceding sections have counterparts in community-based living that are evident and do not need further discussion here. Also, note that all of the quotes about the effects of stigma on connectedness were taken from people living in their own homes, not in nursing homes. Similarly, the discussion that follows on enhancing connectedness will have applicability across the full range of living environments.

Enhancing Connectedness

Just as the domain of connectedness is challenged by personal, operational, and physical barriers, all three types of transformation also can be employed to restore it.

Personal Transformation

Connectedness is primarily about the *interpersonal* domain, and that is where I focus most of my discussion. However, one point I will make about the *intrapersonal* aspect is that we must reexamine the ways in which the stigma of dementia challenges people's identity, and subsequently our willingness and ability to connect with them in a meaningful way. The quotes from the first section of this chapter, as well as the content of the previous chapter, give us a solid foundation for beginning to shift our own perspective.

A more enlightened mindset recognizes the value of connection and inclusion, blurring the lines between "us" and "them" to help move from stigmatization to normalization. Robert Simpson offers this advice:

> In my mind, one of the most important things you could do for me to make me feel comfortable in a group of people is to include me. Not so much by asking questions, unless you are willing to help me answer them (which I would appreciate), but by including me in your smiles and eye contact. (Simpson & Simpson, 1999, p. 134)

As emphasized in *Dementia Beyond Drugs*, much of the basis for a successful interaction lies in being fully "present," and in the intention that one brings to the encounter. Or stated another way:

> Approach the person with forgetfulness as if you were about to enter the unknown, a sacred space. Communication is not only about content. It is also—sometimes most of all—about feelings. (Shabahangi & Szymkiewicz, 2008, p. 71)

Expanding upon this quote from a conversation we had, Dr. Nader Shabahangi reminded me that Nietzsche once said, "Without forgetting, it is quite impossible to live at all." Shabahangi used that quote to explain his philosophy that the secret to making a successful connection with a forgetful person requires that we temporarily enter a realm of forgetting as well. We must forget the past and future in order to free our minds of intrusive thoughts and be with the person in the present moment. We must also forget our own identity, for the imposition of our ego and our reality prevents us from truly hearing the person and understanding his perspective.

In *Dementia Beyond Drugs*, I devoted a good deal of discussion to the basics of *interpersonal* interaction, particularly in Chapters 9 and 10. I will not repeat the contents of the book, but will emphasize that the information in those chapters is critical to positive engagement and, as we will discuss later, to enhancing security and autonomy as well. For readers not familiar with those chapters, I would recommend reviewing them at this juncture.

Many of the concepts discussed in those chapters are very basic and may not seem worth mentioning. Nevertheless, a visit to the vast majority of living environments will find those "basics" largely missing in regular interactions, due to our tendency to focus on time and tasks instead of people. I believe that if people living with dementia were supported by dedicated, consistent care partners who used those basic interpersonal skills in all encounters, the majority of episodes of distress would be prevented without any further interventions or transformative work. It is that important.

Beyond those suggestions, however, I would like to discuss a few other points that go beyond the information contained in *Dementia Beyond Drugs*. In pages 165–167 of the book, I discuss various aspects of conversing in a way that preserves self-esteem. Those pages contain several pointers on the "fine art of conversation" with a person who is forgetful.

In my seminars, I have taken this a bit further by encouraging participants to "speak like a sports interviewer." I have long felt that sports interviews are rather odd, because the reporters rarely ask questions. If the Yankees lose a baseball game and Derek Jeter comes limping off the field, head bowed, a reporter might approach him and say, "Well, Derek, it was a pretty rough day out there." Then he would point the microphone at the player's mouth and await a response without actually having posed a proper question.

I used to be amused at this technique, but realized that it is actually an excellent way to converse with a person who is forgetful. Normally, when we converse with each other, we often do it in the form of questions: "How was your weekend? How was that new restaurant you went to? What did you have to eat?" and so on. This is fine for people with good memories, but for the forgetful, it is a string of demands for information they cannot retrieve. The result is a feeling of failure and low self-esteem after searching for so many answers and coming up empty. It is often much better to simply make an observation and give the person space to fill in as he pleases. This way, the person may add a little or a lot of detail—the choice and content are up to him. Any answer can be the "right" answer because *he* sets the parameters, not us.

Robert Simpson (Simpson & Simpson, 1999) agrees:

> Don't ask me—tell me! Then I don't feel pressure. If someone says, "Do you remember . . . ?" or "Do you know who I am?" the pressure makes me panic. (p. 44)

Of course, an important correlate to this is not to diminish the person's response if he does not remember things exactly the way we do. It is rarely so important that it needs correction, and as we will discuss shortly, a focus on the "facts" may cause us to miss the real message. I often chide my audiences that "you don't need to have dementia to remember things differently; you only need to be in a romantic relationship!"

A second concept around enhancing communication is the "word palette," which is espoused by Daniella Greenwood, Strategy and Innovation Manager for the Arcare Australia organization (D. Greenwood, personal communication, September 2, 2013). The basic concept is as follows:

> Just as each artist uses a palette of colors unique to her or his style of painting, each person develops a "palette" of language that reflects her or his background, culture, education, and worldview. As the person's life with dementia evolves, that palette may retain many of its original "colors," but the process over time may also affect word choices and language to some extent.
>
> An essential tool of good communication is to use one's knowledge of the person to discover her "word palette" in order to learn how best to understand and be understood throughout changes in her memory and word-finding ability. It goes without saying that regular contact and deep knowing are required to develop this skill to the fullest.

This is not to say that we should speak in crude caricature that is not true to our own language, if the person comes from a different background. Rather, care partners should understand the word choices that will best convey the ideas they wish to express, rather than using phrases that could confuse or even insult a person who is used to a different style of communication.

The story related in Chapter 3 about the retired doctor who was being addressed by his first name and not being involved in decision making is an example of a person from a certain educational and occupational background responding negatively to conversation that did not acknowledge his style of interaction and language.

In my conversation with Greenwood about this concept, she gave the example of a woman she visited regularly who formerly held a university academic post. When spoken to in language that reflected her own word palette, she sat straight in her chair and was more engaging and attentive than when spoken to as a typical person with advanced dementia might be addressed. Enhanced connectedness through recognition of identity—once again the two domains act in concert.

Sometimes the effect of dementia is to cause a person to choose words or phrases that may not make sense to a stranger, but whose meaning can only be inferred by knowing the person well. Thus, people with more advanced language difficulties may express discomfort, fear, sadness, or anger with a novel palette of colors. The gifted care partner will use her insights to look beyond the words and understand the new colors that the person is using to paint a representation of her current thoughts and feelings.

A third area of enlightened communication expands on the quote from Christine Bryden that I mentioned in the first section of this chapter—that people with dementia make a journey "from cognition, through emotion, and finally into spirit." As care partners, our minds remain firmly anchored in the "first world" of cognition, so our typical response to a person's statement tends to focus on the facts or logic of the comment. As a result, we often fail to recognize the underlying emotion or symbolism that is the true nature of the comment. By validating the emotion expressed, and exploring those feelings in a nonjudgmental way, we can obtain much more information about the need that is being communicated.

Fazio (2008) echoes this idea:

> [People living with dementia] may retreat from an *intellectual existence* to a place of inner riches and spiritual freedom. In a sense, they can experience a reawakening or a return to a more genuine and authentic existence. They can connect on both a deeper and simpler level— heart to heart or soul to soul rather than mind to mind. Those who care for persons with Alzheimer's have the same ability, but may not necessarily realize it. Caregivers too often overlook these powerful, yet subtle connections because they become preoccupied with frustrations of loss and focus on what the person can no longer do. (p. 107)

Kitwood (1997) also argues that such communication should "Take us out of our customary patterns of over-busyness, hypercognitivism and extreme talkivity, into a way of being in which emotion and feeling are given a much larger place." (p. 5) An example of such a communication mismatch can be seen in the responses commonly given to the statement, "I want to go home." In the nursing home or assisted living setting, this comment is often answered by attempts to reassure the person that she lives here now, that *this* is her new home. Some will go as far as to explain that the old home has been sold, or that she is too frail, sick, or dependent to go back there to live. All of these responses miss the larger point.

For a person making the journey from cognition into emotion, the statement rarely means, "I want to go to the house at 35 Elm Street with the green shutters and the rose garden in the front." What it more often means is, "The place I am in right now does not have the *attributes* that feel like home to me." And those missing attributes generally reside in the domains of well-being.

The person may actually be saying, "I don't feel well known, a sense of belonging, secure, or in control in my present surroundings." Or perhaps, "The things I am doing here are not meaningful to me." When you look at the comment from this perspective, it becomes easy to see why a response such as "This is where you live now" is not comforting to people. After all, they just told you they do not feel right in this place, and your response was that this is where they need to stay.

A person may even express the desire to go home while living in her own home. Instead of simply concluding that "she is so confused that she doesn't even know where she is anymore," this insight helps us to find the real meaning of the comment and enhance those aspects of well-being that have suffered as a result of the intrinsic and extrinsic forces at work in any living environment.

During a seminar I facilitated in London, U.K., one of the participants shared a moving story that speaks to this topic:

> A woman living at a nursing home repeatedly asked for her mother, who was long deceased. The care partners gave her a variety of responses, from distractions to small untruths about where her mother might be, even trying on occasion to gently break the news of her mother's death. Nothing helped.
>
> Finally, a care partner was attending to the woman one day and the woman repeated her request for her mother. She said to the woman, "I am sorry you miss your mother. What would she do if she were here now?"
>
> Without hesitation, the woman responded, "She would love me." This was a stark and sobering statement about the low degree of affection and connectedness she was feeling from the staff. This insight helped the staff to learn how to provide

her with the tender care that she had been missing (and asking for in her own symbolic way).

I explore this topic further and share more powerful stories in Chapter 7 ("Meaning").

The "Being" Connection

In *Dementia Beyond Drugs*, I discuss the concepts of *doing* and *being*, and describe how our focus on tasks and skills leads us to value doing activities while underrecognizing people's need to simply *be*. I recall talking about this concept with co-workers at St. John's Home in Rochester, and one of the nursing assistants made this astute observation:

> For a lot of the people living here, it must be like sitting on the edge of a highway and everyone is rushing back and forth like cars on the highway. And no one takes the time to break out of the flow of traffic and just stop and connect with you for a few minutes.

To restate a point from *Dementia Beyond Drugs*, for people who do less, remember less, or say less, the value of doing activities decreases while the value of simply connecting becomes paramount. Because our systems of care reflect society's tendency to value doing over being, we often fail to understand that the best response to a person's distress is usually not one of more activity. Sitting together with little or no conversation, holding a hand, sharing space and time can be our best responses. This is another example of our need to resist the paradigm that the only valuable components of care are those that can be easily measured.

There is much more that can be said about the value of being. One of the best sources is *Inside Alzheimer's* by Nancy Pearce (2011), who echoes my thoughts about the importance of care partners being mindful and present whenever engaging people living with dementia:

> Deep inner silence is constantly challenged during our interactions with a person who has dementia, and yet, in my experience, it is essential. When I focus on calming my mind, I open more readily and fully to communicating through the heart. . . . Only in such inner silence can I put aside my perception of my world, enter the world of the person with dementia and fully 'listen' to what he is communicating at the moment. This listening in silence is not passivity; it is whole, attentive presence. (p. 117)

I will finish this discussion with two challenges for professional care partners. One commonly expressed barrier to building relationships and getting to know individuals is lack of time. I commonly respond by asking, "How long does it take for you to help someone bathe, or get dressed?" The truth is that the time spent during hands-on care is a perfect opportunity to build relationships. The task will still be accomplished; the only difference is the degree of interaction and intent that occurs during the task.

Beyond that, however, I have another challenge for professional staff in relationship building, which requires a small investment of time, but will pay large dividends. For those who work in long-term care settings, ask this question of yourselves and your co-workers: How often do you enter a person's room or approach him when you don't have something you want him to do at that moment?

We like to think that we are person-centered, yet most, if not all, of our interactions revolve around tasks (dressing, bathing, medications, or transporting to meals, activities, etc.). How often do we sit for a few minutes and talk with a person when we have no other agenda? We often describe people as guarded, suspicious, or downright paranoid; yet how would you feel if a friend or co-worker only spoke to you when she wanted a favor? True relationship building requires a commitment to the person that is not simply based on performing tasks. An occasional brief visit when no other task is being performed can have a striking effect on someone's demeanor.

Touching on Intimacy

One hot topic that is often raised when discussing people with cognitive illness is that of intimacy and romantic relationships. Many concerns arise from the person's expressed desire for this type of connectedness. A wide variety of issues on this topic could be presented here (and some were addressed in *Dementia Beyond Drugs*). For the purposes of this chapter, I would like to focus on challenging our own preconceptions about two areas: (1) the meaning of intimacy and (2) the ability of people living with dementia to form intimate relationships.

An obvious preconception that commonly arises is that intimacy means sex. Our society's hypersexual focus, fueled by advertising and other media, often leads us to assume that certain words or actions denote a desire for sexual activity, when this is often not the case.

In her memoir about caring for her husband, Lela Knox Shanks (1999) makes the following observation:

> In its broadest terms, intimacy was best defined for me in an article about Laurel Van Ham, a family practice counselor who defined intimacy as "knowing the internal reality of another person and letting that person know your internal reality, all in an atmosphere of unconditional acceptance." . . . Culture, she said, "messes us up because we have this phrase that 'two people were intimate' and we mean sex . . . aside from sexual closeness, intimacy can be spiritual, intellectual or aesthetic—like watching a sunset with a neighbor, enjoying a ballet with a co-worker, being part of a prayer circle . . . " (pp. 147–148)

Shanks also mentions that between the choices of sexual intercourse versus total abstinence "sexuality can be experienced and appreciated in its broadest sense: the physical closeness of hugging, kissing, stroking, caressing, snuggling, touching. Persons with [Alzheimer's disease] continue to be human beings despite their mental deterioration and may thus have an ongoing need for this kind of physical intimacy" (p. 148).

Taylor (2007) agrees:

> My relationship with my spouse, my family, and my friends has broadened and in some ways deepened. We spend more time really being together. We talk more, we hug more, we cry more, we laugh more and harder and longer together. . . .
>
> As I became still older, I was finally able to place sex as a part of intimacy, rather than vice versa. There are no pills that increase or decrease my desire to be intimate. (pp. 169–170)

Thus, even though many couples have an active sexual life, there are many forms of intimacy that they share, and many of those persist beyond the couple's desire or ability to continue sexual relations. These aspects of connectedness are frequently disrupted when one half of a couple moves to a long-term care environment, as many countries' regulations do not support the couple living together if they do not require the same level of care.

Added to this separation is the medicalized living environment that teaches care partners to interact with clinical detachment and to be very reserved regarding touch. The result is that both the personal and the emotional closeness that had been experienced at home have been suddenly withdrawn, coincident with the feelings of confusion, displacement, and insecurity that such a move often produces. In this situation, many people living with dementia reach out for human contact. Because their ability to communicate their need is often impaired, they may reach out in ways that feel inappropriate or unwelcome to those around them. Understanding what lies beneath these expressions is the first step to finding a solution.

The key is to create connectedness in ways that are healthy and nurturing. In part, this may involve creating more opportunities where affectionate but appropriate touch can be used in daily interactions—a hug upon greeting, a reassuring pat on the shoulder, or the gentle touch of a hand on someone's arm.

One situation where this knowledge can provide insight is the not uncommon occurrence of a person climbing into another person's bed at night. In most cases, this is less due to the desire for sexual activity than re-creating the long-time experience of sleeping next to a loved one. I have heard of several situations where a body pillow in the bed provided a feeling of close contact that promoted a sense of security at night and removed the person's need to find the contact elsewhere.

Sarah Rowan (2011), who speaks extensively about caring for her late husband, Joseph, recalled a time when he lived in a nursing home and was regularly climbing into bed with a woman who lived down the hall. Sarah recognized this need for physical closeness that Joseph had lost in moving to the home, and she was able to support this connection, which seemed to benefit both parties. She recalled one occasion when Joseph had positioned himself in such a way that the woman was in danger of falling out of the bed. She repositioned him and later remarked, "I never thought I would see the day when I would be helping my husband get into bed with another woman!"

Another preconception we need to challenge is our view of the ability of people living with dementia to enter into relationships with others. Of course, we have an obligation to help people who are severely affected to make safe choices. And there is a wide spectrum of situations that demands individualized approaches. But as with other aspects of life, the stigma starts early, and we need to be aware of the power of the label "dementia."

It strikes me that there are many people in our society who make incredibly bad choices regarding their love lives (insert the names of many an entertainer, politician, or athlete here). And yet, we never question their right to make such choices as competent adults. Not so for people who have acquired a label such as "Alzheimer's" or "dementia."

I recently asked Christine Bryden to share her own experiences with me in this regard (personal communication, September 8, 2013). Christine met her husband Paul 3 years after she was diagnosed. Now married for over 14 years, they have had a strong and healthy relationship, and Paul has been a great support for Christine as she lives with cognitive disability. But how did that go for them at the outset?

Christine had divorced her first husband before the time of her diagnosis (in 1995 at age 46). Initially, she was devastated by the news of her illness, but through the support of friends and family, she began to reclaim her hope for a positive life, however long it might last.

In 1998, Christine decided that it would be better if she could find someone with whom she could share her life. She approached an introductions agency to search for a potential companion. She felt that the agency would help her to sort out people with common interests, and would be a safer way to meet someone; however, she was careful not to tell the agency about her diagnosis, as she was certain that they would drop her. "The stigma of dementia is that we have lost our ability to think, to have insight, to make decisions. We are also thought to be already in the last stages, so why bother being in a relationship with us?"

The agency soon contacted Christine with an interested party, who turned out to be Paul. He sounded delightful and they set up a time and place to meet. Paul was charming; he brought her a bouquet of flowers and a fancy picnic lunch for them to share by a lake in a nearby park. As enjoyable as the afternoon was, Christine felt it was dishonest to continue without "coming clean," so she told Paul about her diagnosis. To her surprise, Paul told Christine about his father, who had lived with dementia and died a few years earlier, and he continued to be interested in pursuing a relationship with her.

The romance quickly blossomed, but some trials were ahead as they "went public." Both Christine and Paul fell prey to the effects of stigma. Christine was quizzed by friends and family alike, with the implication that "surely she is not able to think clearly about her choices at this time." She realized that this reaction was motivated by love and a concern to protect her, but, nevertheless, "reactions were on the whole negative."

Paul found himself being grilled by Christine's advocates, to be sure his motives were pure; once again, the stigma led people to wonder, "'Why is he interested in her? Is it about money?' (not that I had much)." Paul also faced questions from his own family that reflect societal stigmas about dementia:

"Paul needed to reassure his family . . . that he was making a wise choice, that he was happy, and that I was not 'demented.'"

Paul acquitted himself very well, first with family and friends in Australia, then with Christine's family members in the United Kingdom and Belgium. It took some time for his pending divorce to be granted, so he officially proposed a year later, in July 1999, and they were married in August. Their families attended, as did members of Christine's dementia support group, and it was "a lovely celebratory atmosphere."

Now, nearly 15 years on, Christine reflects that a major support in helping them to prevail was their shared Christian faith, which "gives Paul the confidence and patience to cope with my changing needs." Paul's work in the diplomatic corps also enabled Christine to travel and connect with kindred spirits around the world, and an international support network was formed.

Looking back on their loving marriage, Christine adds these words of wisdom: "It is all too easy for people with dementia to be devalued by society, by the stigma that surrounds us. The stigma in society in turn creates a stigma within us, as we begin to respond to the web of misconception and discrimination around us. . . .

"Human beings are created to be in relationship, and without connectedness within society they lose an important source of meaning in life."

So whether through a romantic relationship or other forms of social engagement, connectedness creates meaning. We will explore that concept further in Chapter 7.

Although Christine Bryden's story is noteworthy, one might argue that her level of function in the community put her in a different position to enter into a relationship than a person living in a nursing home. But the needs of people in long-term care do not disappear, and it is important to avoid the all-or-none approach to this issue as well.

One organization known for its frank and carefully planned approach to this topic is the Hebrew Home at Riverdale, in the Bronx borough of New York City. Their efforts to address this important need dates back to 1995, when their first policy was drafted. Updated in 2013, their sexual expression policy reaffirms "the older adult's right to engage in sexual activity, as long as there is consent among those involved," as "demonstrated by the words and/or affirmative actions of an older adult" (Dessel & Ramirez, 2013a, p. 2).

The policy explicitly states that adults living with dementia are included in the guidelines, and that such contact may occur between two residents of the home, or between a resident and a visitor who meets the guidelines. The policy also provides for the possession of legal, explicit media, as well as an obligation to ensure that private space is available for any such activity.

In order to create reasonable safeguards against the potential for abuse or nonconsensual contact, there is an accompanying document that defines appropriate and inappropriate contact and provides a procedure for assessing consent (Dessel & Ramirez, 2013b). The latter evaluates the person's ability to express consent, the person's ability to appreciate the sexual activity, and the expression of "personal quality of life choices in the here and now." A series of suggested questions and observations acts as a guide.

All activity needs to occur within legal and health parameters, and a relevant family member or legal representative is involved when there is a diagnosis of a cognitive impairment. However, the clear and consistent expression of consent of an individual is to be respected, regardless of the personal views of relatives or staff. It would be beneficial for all homes to review this policy and begin a discussion about creating similar guidelines for their organization, residents, and staff.

Operational Transformation

I have made the argument for enhancing connectedness through dedicated care partnerships in all living environments, and have presented several theoretical points to bolster that view. Consider the real-life initiative of an organization in Australia and the success they achieved, even in the earliest weeks of the initiative.

Arcare operates 22 residential homes in Victoria and Queensland, Australia, serving nearly 2,000 people with various care needs, as well as providing home care services to nearby communities. Among their residences are a number of "sensitive care" environments for people living with dementia. Daniella Greenwood, Strategy and Innovation Manager for the organization, recognized early on the critical importance of dedicated staffing for these environments, but Arcare had not yet adopted this strategy. Charged with bringing Arcare's service quality to the next level, Greenwood began with an action study using an appreciative inquiry approach. She held a series of focus groups and individual interviews with a total of 80 elders, family members, and staff, from both residential and community care.

The study identified four main areas of focus: (1) *connections*, which encompass relationships, community, and "beyond the physical"; (2) *recognition*, which encompasses seeing the person, seeing loss, and seeing beyond words; (3) *partnerships*, which encompass broadening the circle of partners and enabling partnerships; and (4) *possibility*, which encompasses two paired themes of growth and purpose, and fun and joy. (As with the Murray Alzheimer Research and Education Program [MAREP] "Living Life through Leisure" study mentioned in Chapter 2, note how the seven domains of well-being are so nicely enmeshed in these areas identified by the participants.)

In the area of connections, several of the participants' comments highlight the value of this domain for all involved (Greenwood, 2012, p. 13):

> A young carer . . . just made me completely relaxed, and my daughter too, and we both look at him as a personal friend now. (Elder)

> If you know that one person has that little connection, and they're the ones that have that sort of little vibe with your loved one, yeah, absolutely, you feel real peace of mind. (Family member)

> Just knowing that you have connected, end of story, it doesn't matter if they say a word or not, just seeing that smile on their face when you walk in the room says it all and you can walk away thinking, well, I've done my job. (Staff member)

Additional comments reflected upon the difficulty that elders and their families faced in needing to develop familiarity and trust anew when staff were moved to another living area. One person stated that many of the needs of a loved one often "can't be captured on a form" (p. 13). Another stated that families had an important role in helping their loved ones to make new friends and build community in the new living environment.

Two other quoted comments from the survey lend support to points made earlier in this chapter. On the topic of integrated living, one elder said: "I think we should all live with (people with dementia), and we get to accept each other, and that's the way it's been where we are, we all accept our little problems, and everyone is very understanding" (p. 15). And on the topic of relationship building, a family member said, "people need to have a relationship with my mum, a one-on-one relationship, a rapport, and not just doing things for her" (p. 15).

Based on this important input, Greenwood began a process of transitioning the homes to embrace dedicated staffing. She quickly recognized that not all people working in these environments were ideally suited for this initiative, so all hands-on employees who wanted to work in these areas went through a reapplication process. Those who did not wish to, or who were not ultimately accepted, were allowed to move to other areas of the organization. The initial response to the initiative was overwhelming—a credit to Greenwood for convincing people of the importance of a concept that so often is met with resistance from hands-on staff and leadership alike.

The results were immediate and striking, as a video made for the corporate leaders attests (Arcare, 2013). Very early in the initiative, one family member offered this comment: "For the first time in three years I can sleep in . . . because I know exactly who is with Irene that morning . . . and I trust them."

After only 6 weeks, staff members were noted to be spending more time in meaningful engagement with the elders, without sacrificing completion of tasks. One care partner spoke about the awkward experiences he had encountered previously through rotating assignments, when people did not know him and were guarded and questioning of his motives when he approached. He then expressed his appreciation for the new initiative because the elders were warm, relaxed, and welcoming through their deeper knowledge of him as a regular care partner.

The most powerful testimonial came from a man whose mother had recently passed away. He described the love and care provided by the staff, and how they spent time with her "talking about things that they knew mattered to Mum. That dedicated staff over the last few weeks with Mum, and me, made all the difference." He went on to extol the strong feeling of community and family that the initiative created; he described his mother's passing as "an achievement" and added, in a voice choked with emotion, "It was a blessing to be part of it" (Arcare, 2013).

As Arcare moved to dedicated staff assignments, they also noticed significant clinical changes early on. In the first 6 months at one of their first communities to implement dedicated assignments, they noted a 70% drop in chest infections, compared with both the previous 6-month period and with the same season of the previous year (Greenwood, personal communication, October 26, 2013). This could well be related to fewer staff coming into contact with the elders, as the roster dropped from 48 care partners to 26, all working at least three shifts per week. The number of different care partners supporting each elder on day and evening shifts combined over a 30-day period dropped from 28 to 4! Greenwood also noted a 100% drop in pressure sores during this period, which could possibly be related to better quality personal care by knowing staff, as well as proactive reduction of other risk factors.

This outcome echoes that of a large urban nursing home in California, which implemented a variety of culture change strategies, a cornerstone of which was the switch to dedicated staff assignments (Farrell & Frank, 2007). Outcomes included a decrease in high-risk pressure ulcers from 25% to 11%, and a decrease in low-risk pressure ulcers from 4.5% to 0%. (Other outcomes reported by Farrell and Frank included a decrease in annualized nursing assistant turnover from 94% to 38%, a decrease in licensed nurse turnover from 43% to 11%, and an increase in nursing home occupancy from 82% to 94%.)

Another important result of Arcare's dedicated staff initiative was a 100% reduction in family concerns lodged through their official complaint system. While many of these outcomes are difficult to quantify in economic terms, their impact—clinical, relational, ethical, *and* financial—is certainly significant.

Consistency in relationships is equally important in community settings, but beyond the realm of professional home care staff, not all members of one's social network have the skill or desire to connect in this way, often due to lack of education, or stigma-based fears. While education can help overcome many barriers, recognizing the limits of individual family members and friends helps create a web of support that suits each person's strengths.

Shanks (1999) navigated this terrain beautifully in creating a network of support for her husband, Hughes:

> Though the greatest need of the caregiver is respite service, not every member of our support system is physically, mentally or emotionally equipped to provide personal hands-on care. . . . We cannot give what we do not have, but one who cares about the patient and the caregiver can always do something—and we have received a variety of unusual and unexpected kinds of support. For example, when Hughes was in the beginning stage of his disease, his friend, Dean, volunteered to screen in our front porch; he and his wife, Sonja, thought Hughes might better enjoy sitting there if it was made private. Little did I know then how much this locked, screened porch would help me years later as a safe and secure area where Hughes could walk or sit while I worked nearby at my computer. (p. 111)

The preceding quote shows that connectedness can be created in many ways, by tapping into a person's unique abilities. One recurring theme of this book will be a call to avoid seeing any aspect of life and care for people with dementia in black-and-white, or all-or-none terms.

Reimagining Support Groups

Another operational change that is too commonly overlooked in the community involves creating connectedness *between* people living with dementia. The majority of available support groups are either designed for family care partners or for groups that include people living with the diagnosis in combination with family members. While both formats serve a useful purpose, there is a benefit to enabling people with dementia to connect without moderation by families or professionals, which is often unseen when stigma clouds our view.

A colleague once attended a presentation on a "Memory Café" program that was highly touted as an important social outlet for people living with dementia. But the presentation referred only to the inclusion of people with dementia in tandem with family members. After the session, my colleague approached the presenter and asked, "Suppose I had a diagnosis of dementia and had not yet revealed this, even to close friends and family members. If I wanted some support, would I be able to attend the café?" The rather measured response was, "Well, we might arrange to have you come sit in on a session; but we really would prefer that you attend with a family member."

Just as Ed Voris found when he went alone to local support chapters for information, the common view still exists that "you cannot benefit from our services unless you have someone without dementia at your side to explain it all to you." Once again, the label makes us devolve into all-or-none thinking.

O'Connor (2002) found that the family support groups she studied tended to focus heavily on helping the care partner to cope and did not provide any degree of empowerment for those living with dementia. And Bartlett and O'Connor (2010) quote a 2008 study by Linda Clare of support groups designed for people with dementia, in which the primary dynamic consisted of the facilitator addressing each person in dialogue, without also facilitating meaningful interaction between the participants. Clearly, many of the counselors who convene such groups need to reframe their view of what can be accomplished in such peer support groups and improve their skills at facilitating interaction and dialogue among the participants.

However, while some facilitation and structure might be needed at the outset, there are many reasons why people living with cognitive disabilities can benefit from meeting each other without family members present. They have a unique understanding of their situation that is often hard to explain to those who have not experienced it. They often sense feelings and connect at levels that others do not appreciate. The pace and content of the discussion is dictated by them and not the "well other," and the likelihood of a family member dominating or coloring the conversation is eliminated. And like family care partners who prefer to meet separately at times, they may need their own space to vent frustrations and fears without worrying about how their comments might affect their loved ones.

Enter Dr. Richard Taylor, who looked back upon his own grief-stricken reaction to his diagnosis and realized that something was missing in his support system:

> As I've traveled around speaking to other people who have dementia, I've stumbled across a common theme with them. Their anxiety and their depression . . . and their sense of being abnormal was reduced when they met other people with dementia, when they were in the same room with kindred spirits. . . .
>
> Now you can read all the websites you want to . . . and you can go to all the self-help groups, and you can talk to all the professionals, but what you won't have is a sense of normality for yourself. As a matter of fact, it just made me feel more abnormal when I found all the information about how I was different from other people and how my life would be different. (Taylor, 2012)

To this end, Taylor formed the nonprofit organization Dementia Support Networks USA (following the lead of similar organizations, such as Dementia Advocacy and Support Network International, which Christine Bryden helped spearhead in 2000). Through his work, Taylor has advocated for the establishment of local gatherings where people, particularly early after their diagnosis, can meet socially with others to share their experiences. Family members can help promote these, particularly by organizing the dates and providing transportation. But the primary purpose is for "like-minded" people to connect and discuss the issues they face in daily life.

Taylor calls these "Hello Dinners," because he feels that more often people with dementia are attending "Goodbye Dinners," where the focus is on their deficits and their decline. Indeed, many traditional support groups, whether for family members alone or with their loved one, tend to focus on the deficits, losses, and problems encountered and, therefore, dwell on the stigma, disease, and person who is fading away. The Hello Dinner serves to normalize the person, not only for her own benefit, but often for her family members as well, by having each participant with dementia provide witness to, thereby preserving each other's enduring personhood.

To help people in their greatest moments of need, Taylor feels that doctors should keep a list of their patients diagnosed with dementia who are willing to engage others who are newly diagnosed. He favors an open-ended agenda for these meetings: "Remember, the goal is not to give people more information; the goal is to give them a witness to support a feeling that they're okay" (Taylor, 2012).

Where an established network for such informal dinners does not exist, community organizations can help fill the gap by understanding that support groups by and for people living with dementia are as important as the traditional group meetings they regularly offer. The resulting benefits will help people move beyond the stigmas that have dictated the ways in which people living with dementia can or should be engaged.

I had the privilege of sitting in on a support group meeting for people living with dementia and their care partners that Taylor facilitated. We were speaking for the Alzheimer's Resource of Alaska in Anchorage, and he was invited to be the guest facilitator at one of their scheduled meetings.

Taylor has the dual advantage of being a psychologist and a person living with Alzheimer's. The meeting went far beyond the scheduled time limit, but no one moved a muscle in the jam-packed room. Taylor's ability to connect with others who share the perspective of living with dementia, combined with his sensitivity to all that was said (and not said), wove an intricate web of connectedness—between care partners, between those living with dementia, and, ultimately, between each pair that attended. It was an inspirational example of how one can facilitate mixed support groups through diverse engagement and inclusion of all.

Physical Transformation

How do we design for enhanced connectedness? Part of this was addressed in the last chapter (which discussed supporting one's evolving identity), because connectedness involves preserving contact with all that makes up the individual. While Chapter 3 addressed many of the trappings of the physical environment with respect to enhancing identity, this section focuses on some of the larger design features that connect people.

In the community, maximizing connectedness includes the need for safe, facilitated engagement outside the home. With the aging of our population, much work is being done to create "age-friendly" communities; with some further consideration, these communities can become more "dementia-friendly" as well (see also Chapter 11).

Part of this lies in the physical design of our communities. Neighborhoods that have sidewalks, adequate lighting, and places to stop and rest will enable people to engage more readily outside of their own home. Careful attention to signage that provides adequate wayfinding cues and pathways that accommodate walkers and wheelchairs will help people stay connected as well. There need to be places available to engage the person outside the home, with reasonable proximity and accessibility.

In addition to physical changes, changes in infrastructure (public transport, informal and formal gathering places, etc.) can help to facilitate community connectedness. Many communities are also educating their residents about people with dementia, so that the local shop owner or bus driver will have improved awareness and skills in engaging people living with dementia who may need assistance.

These are only a few examples from a rapidly emerging movement that reaches far beyond what can be discussed here. There are many projects being launched around the world, from large international groups such as the World Health Organization to local community initiatives.

In long-term living environments, size and scale are of primary importance. As a rule, congregate living environments are larger and hold more people than one's own home. We have discussed how the size of a living environment creates functional barriers to connectedness. But less apparent are the psychological barriers it creates.

Environmental gerontologist Dr. Emi Kiyota (2011) has a basic rule about creating a feeling of home versus an institutional feeling: *Size trumps décor*. In other words: homes are cozy; institutions are not. A dining room may have beautiful furniture and decorations, but if there are ten tables seating four people each, it will feel institutional, whereas a smaller room without the fancy décor and a single communal table will feel more like home.

Why? The answer lies in connectedness. When you share a space with people you cannot easily see, hear, or otherwise engage, you lose that feeling of connectedness; such a loss is a hallmark of institutional living. Smaller environments should always be the goal, whether through individual small houses or households within a larger structure. When renovation dollars are short, using minor physical changes to break up larger areas into smaller ones can be accomplished without huge expenditures. A door or half-wall across a hallway or dividers in large communal areas can help people to focus on their immediate surroundings and not be distracted by sounds or sights beyond their immediate area of engagement.

Keep in mind that such physical changes require operational shifts for optimal effect. Breaking up large living areas into smaller ones only works if staff members respect those boundaries and avoid passing through or even entering them unless they have a consistent relationship with the people who live there and a purpose for entering at that time.

Finally, design can be used to influence behavior—in this case, the word *behavior* applies equally or more so to those who support the people living there. Gojikara Village, a multigenerational village in southern Japan, uses a variety of physical and operational features to help enhance connectedness and other domains of well-being. In the village, the care partners who work with the elders must park their cars in a lot situated away from the home, and follow a winding wooded path to the entrance. This helps people to relax and slow their minds and bodies to a pace that is more congruent with that of the elders they serve. There is also a limit to the ease of access into buildings for older people; many steps remain in place, so that younger people will engage an elder by helping her up the steps.

An example of an operational shift is the use of the lunchroom at the nursing home in Gojikara. The elders eat at noon and the nursing students are asked to eat at one o'clock, but they are allowed in at noon if they are willing to sit with and assist an elder, thus giving an incentive for fostering engagement. (A similar philosophy is central to the Green House® model, where the versatile staff members not only prepare the meals, but also sit and share them with the elders, rather than going off on a separate meal break.)

Gojikara Village also rents apartments to young professional women at a favorable rate on a floor above elder apartments, to encourage the development of relationships between neighbors of different generations. In these ways, the physical and operational features gently nudge people toward a level of connectedness that is organic and natural, rather than simply mandating relationship-building in some artificial manner.

Lastly, it would be unwise for the reader to jump to the conclusion that designing for connectedness favors the use of shared bedrooms and bathrooms. We need both connectedness and privacy in our lives. We will explore this topic further in the next chapter.

CHAPTER 5

Security

The ache for home lives in all of us, the safe place where
we can go as we are and not be questioned.

—Maya Angelou

The fact is that people are good. Give people affection and
security, and they will give affection and be secure in their
feelings and their behavior.

—Abraham Maslow

Security Defined

Fox et al. (2005) use the following terms to describe the many aspects of the domain of security: "Freedom from doubt, anxiety or fear; safe, certain, assured; having privacy, dignity and respect." Therefore, security is much more than simply an exit alarm system on the door of a nursing home. It reflects one's internal familiarity and comfort with one's surroundings, and it also reflects the ways in which we interact with those in our care.

In fact, a narrow definition of security is an all too common feature of all living environments. Due to the combination of a stigmatized view of individuals living with dementia and a society that views individual risk and responsibility through a very litigious lens, our narrow view of safety actually erodes the overall security of the very people we strive to protect.

In this chapter, we will discuss how our systems of care often serve to validate Franklin Delano Roosevelt's caution that "the only thing we have to fear is fear itself." We will challenge the black-and-white approach that many take in providing security for people with dementia and create a more nuanced view that shows how attention to the many varied dimensions of security just described can create an environment that is safe, but not stifling.

Once again, the ordering of the well-being domains in this book lends itself to a better understanding of how they support each other. Identity and connectedness are the foundation to better care and support, through knowing the individual and cultivating ongoing relationships to create an even deeper, more durable knowing, even for the person who is forgetful.

In Chapter 2, I mentioned that personal transformation of a care environment involves both *intrapersonal* and *interpersonal* aspects. Identity can be seen as the domain mostly served by intrapersonal transformation—changing the way we see people living with dementia. Connectedness is more directly served by interpersonal transformation—changing the ways in which we communicate with and support them.

Just as identity and connectedness interrelate so closely, the same applies to security and autonomy, and this and the following chapter will complement each other in many ways. But both chapters also flow from a deep understanding of the first two domains, because only with careful attention to understanding one's identity and shifting the environment to foster connectedness can we create a fertile environment for security and autonomy to thrive.

In Figure 3, I have created a suggested rendering of the Fox et al. (2005) domains of well-being in a pyramid form resembling that of Maslow's hierarchy of needs (Maslow, 1943). Identity and connectedness form the foundation of the pyramid—the basis for creating all types of well-being. Above them, security and autonomy sit side-by-side, interacting closely with each other and supported by identity and connectedness.

As the following chapters will show, security and autonomy are keys to optimizing meaning and growth, which in turn provide the soil in which joy can thrive. As with Maslow's hierarchy, the lower domains are needed in order for the higher ones to be fully realized. Maslow's ultimate goal of self-actualization correlates well with the attainment of meaning and growth in this framework. The term

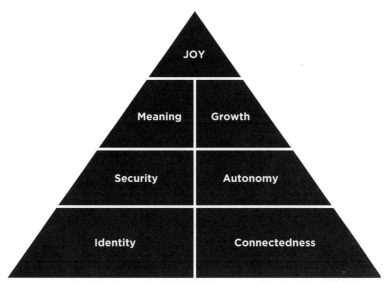

Figure 3. The well-being pyramid illustrates the hierarchy of domains to be addressed for restoring well-being.

self-actualization was first coined by theorist Kurt Goldstein (1939) and later adapted by Maslow to depict what he considered to be the apex of his hierarchy of needs. It refers to the inner drive to fulfill one's maximum potential, "to become everything that one is capable of becoming." (Maslow, 1943, p. 383)

It might be noted that security does not reside on the bottom tier of this rendering, as it does with Maslow's model. This model argues that, for people living with dementia, security is more than simple food and shelter; it requires support from the care environment. Such support can only be fully realized when people are well known and are connected with those around them in a familiar and meaningful way. Although the reader may find other arrangements of the well-being domains equally appealing, I invite you to follow this suggested hierarchy as our discussion of enhancing well-being continues to unfold.

How Dementia Challenges Security

As we saw in the previous two chapters, cognitive changes can erode a sense of emotional security as well as physical safety. But, paradoxically, those who provide care can erode that sense of security further, even when trying to keep the person safe.

Intrinsic Challenges

Beginning with challenges to emotional security, in order to minimize fear and doubt, two features of one's living environment are needed: *familiarity* and *trust*. Imagine for a moment a visit to a carnival fun house. Whether it is the type you walk through or ride through, each one creates "fun frights" by reducing the familiarity of your surroundings and then introducing the unexpected.

So the first rule of the successful fun house is to turn out the lights. Without one's important visual input, the unknown looms larger with each twist and turn. Then people or objects appear or even lurch at you when you least expect it, creating the frights. Even with your guard up, it is difficult not to get spooked.

Now, imagine how it would be if the lights were left on and you were given a schematic that told you exactly what would happen and when. The fear would be greatly diminished or eliminated because all of the elements of surprise and doubt have been removed. The fun house would also be a lot less popular. The point is that increasing *familiarity* is a key to reducing fear and improving one's sense of security.

If the purpose of the fun house is to scare us, why does it elicit squeals of glee, rather than driving everyone away? That is where *trust* comes in. We are willing to subject ourselves to these little surprises, because we know that they are all in fun, and that no true danger awaits us. It is a carnival, after all, so if a figure jumps out of the shadows wielding a knife or chainsaw, our initial shock is tempered by the knowledge that the threat is not real.

But take away the premise of trust and the concept becomes a very different one altogether. Imagine walking down a dark city street or a wooded path and having that same figure jump out, even as a joke. We would not be laughing then. Imagine the feeling a police officer or soldier faces when searching a house for an armed criminal or an enemy combatant. Now the danger is all too real.

The forgetfulness of dementia removes the familiarity of the physical environment, as well as the procedural memory needed to predict what may be happening next. Add to this a lack of trust in those around you to have your best interests at heart (see the "extrinsic challenges" section below), and, as a result, the forgetful person may live in a constant state of anxiety, not knowing where to go or what might come next.

From the standpoint of physical security (safety from bodily harm), other aspects of one's cognitive disability add to the real risk of injury. These include difficulties with wayfinding and spatial orientation, procedural memory, and executive function—effective planning and problem-solving skills. As a result, a person who may explore without boundaries runs the risk of getting lost and disoriented, making a poor decision (such as how to dress on a cold day), or being unable to retrace her steps or figure out how to correct a mistake. These challenges create true risk and are the focus of many of the most vigorous debates around the appropriate care of the person by family members and professionals alike.

Extrinsic Challenges

There are a multitude of extrinsic challenges to security for people who live with dementia. I have allocated the discussions of various challenges to either this section (focusing on long-term care), the section on segregated living environments, or that on community-based living, as the flow of each section dictates. Keep in mind, however, that these challenges do not exclusively reside in one living area alone, and are found to some extent in *all* environments.

Erosion of Trust

As already alluded to, one way in which care partners challenge security is by following practices that erode trust. Without trust, any new or unfamiliar experience brings fear and anxiety; for the very forgetful, every day may be unfamiliar. And the most important determinants of familiarity and trust are the people one encounters every day.

Once again, the shadow cast by rotating care partners looms large. In order to trust, one needs some familiarity with the person—if not a name, then at least a facial recognition or an emotional memory of that face. It takes a certain amount of trust to go with a stranger who wishes to take you to the dining room or to an activity; imagine if that stranger wanted to remove your clothes and bathe you, or help you to the toilet.

But even with dedicated staffing patterns or familiar family members in one's own home, there are many ways in which trust can be eroded. One of the most basic lies in our tone of voice and body language.

In Chapter 4, we discussed how a remarkable attention and sensitivity to nonverbal cues usually accompanies a loss of memory and word-finding skills. A lack of awareness of this can lead the care partner to present herself in a way that magnifies anxiety. We may be preoccupied by a sick child at home, an argument with a co-worker, or a migraine headache; regardless of the cause, presenting oneself with body language that suggests anger, irritation, distraction, or even anxiety of your own may be interpreted by a person with dementia as negative emotion being directed toward him. Often we adopt a posture or tone of voice that we do not even realize is being seen in a negative light.

> I was visiting one of the living areas where I worked at St. John's Home in Rochester, New York. As I passed the lounge, I heard a woman in a recliner chair chanting in a somewhat insistent manner. I didn't know her and could not tell on first listening if she was in distress, or simply self-stimulating with rhythmic speech.
>
> I walked over to her, knelt down beside her, greeted her, introduced myself, and began to engage her in conversation. She clearly was not in a distressed state and instead was very focused, relaxed, and able to engage in simple conversation. As I spoke with her, one of the nursing assistants came into the lounge area. She was taking people down the hall to the dining room for lunch and had come in to get the woman. As she stood watching us converse, she put her hands on her hips, waiting.
>
> The woman, who had been smiling pleasantly, looked over at the aide standing with hands on hips and immediately her voice became gruff and challenging: "What's the matter with you over there, standing so 'high and mighty' like that?" The aide relaxed her posture, apologized, and spoke kindly to the woman, inviting her to lunch. The woman's demeanor followed suit, softening once again.

In this case, a professional who is a superb care partner and is generally well loved adopted an unfortunate pose at the wrong moment, triggering the reaction.

Another part of familiarity, however, is the emotional memory that is created through *repeated* day-to-day contact. Whether positive or negative, the emotional memory created by regular interactions with a particular person is much more durable than the memory required for simply recalling names and dates. If a care partner creates consistently negative interactions, this sort of familiarity can also magnify the challenges of care.

> Psychologist Kort Nygard (2012) tells the story of visiting a woman living with dementia in a nursing home. He went to her

room, knocked on the door, introduced himself, and asked if he could visit. The woman was very friendly and accommodating, and they spent several minutes in pleasant conversation.

While they were conversing, one of the woman's regular care partners walked into the room. The woman looked up and her face immediately flushed red with anger. She jabbed a figure in the staff member's direction, shouting, "You! Get out of here at once!" The staff member saw the woman engaged with Nygard, so she turned and quickly left the room.

Nygard was surprised to have seen such a sudden change in the woman's demeanor. After giving the woman a moment to collect herself, he asked, "What did you think that person was going to do to you?" The woman replied, "I don't know, but it was going to be something bad!"

In this example, there was likely a history of repeated negative interactions, and/or negative body language surrounding the care provided by this staff member. Even though the woman did not remember her name, the staff member had left the indelible impression that whenever she came into the room, "something bad" was likely to occur. (The fact that the staff member walked in without knocking or announcing herself no doubt added further to the woman's eroded sense of security.)

DeBaggio (2002) summarizes a 1999 Johns Hopkins study that highlights the durability of emotional memories:

> Events that create a large emotional impact are usually the ones that are best remembered later. In a new study, researchers explored the connection between emotional memories and the brain's limbic system, which governs the most basic urges and emotions. They showed 10 volunteers a series of pictures: some to elicit strong emotions (both good and bad), some that were emotionally neutral, and some that were intellectually, but not emotionally, interesting. The subjects were monitored by PET scans during the viewing. Four weeks later, they were shown more pictures and asked to identify the ones they had seen . . .
>
> The PET scans revealed more activity in the amygdala when the emotionally powerful images were seen again, and these images were more likely to be recognized four weeks later. These findings suggest that the amygdala is activated by emotional stimuli and that it in turn stimulates the adjacent hippocampus—the major part of the brain involved in long-term memory formation. (pp. 72–73)

The Verbal–Nonverbal Connection

A discussion of nonverbal body language may seem like an unusual place to mention spoken language, but there is a deep connection that reinforces the need to challenge many of the words we commonly use in everyday care. In this book, as well as in *Dementia Beyond Drugs*, I devote careful attention to our choice of words. This is because words that are rooted in a stigmatized view of dementia not only blind us to new insights, but also affect our body language, as well as that of our colleagues.

For example, consider some of the commonly used terms that stigmatize, dehumanize, or blame a person living with dementia who is expressing an unmet need. Terms such as *problem behaviors*, *difficult behaviors*, *acting out*, or simply *being nasty* put the fault squarely on the shoulders of the person in need, thereby casting him in a negative light in our minds.

When we carry this image of the person in our minds, it affects the way we carry ourselves when we approach him and converse with him. The defensiveness or disapproval we feel about the person is what he will read in our faces and our body language, and he will often act angry or defensive as a result of the signals we are projecting. This creates another self-fulfilling prophecy—we expect the person to be "difficult," and our approach ensures that he will respond that way, thus proving the point in our minds. (This cycle does not require that a person have cognitive limitations; a similar cycle of negativity can also happen with co-workers, friends, or even family members when we approach them with a certain expectation.)

The additional danger of using such language (whether spoken or written in medical records, care plans, or other documents) is that these negative labels create the same negative imagery in the minds of others who hear or read our words. They may also approach the person with those thoughts in mind, and he will be subjected to a barrage of negativity throughout the day and night. His trust in those around him is eroded, and therefore his sense of security. Assigning the label of "behavior problem" to someone, therefore, makes him feel less secure, feeds his lack of trust, and ensures that he will, in fact, become a problem! How much of the "challenging behavior" that we experience is actually created or inflamed by our own challenging behavior and words? (I will share a surprisingly simple guideline for word choices in the Enhancing Security section later in this chapter.)

Privacy, Dignity, and Respect

Our working definition of security also encompasses "privacy, dignity, and respect," and the interpersonal environment frequently erodes these as well. In long-term care settings, the first challenge to privacy comes in the form of a shared bedroom and bathroom for a large proportion of our elders. Such rooms are assigned as available; those who occupy them have no input as to who their roommate might be. Beds are often separated by a thin "privacy curtain," a laughable name because it provides little to none.

The typical bathroom often does not have a solid door; instead there is an accordion door, or even another "privacy curtain." Not only is the door less solid than one might prefer, but the bathroom itself is usually situated right by the door to the hallway outside the room. This is certainly an accommodation for efficiency of staff assistance, but the proximity of the toilet to a busy public thoroughfare reduces a person's sense of ease even further.

Added to the lack of structural privacy is the lack of privacy caused by workers coming and going without respecting boundaries of the living space as belonging to the person living there. When we see the environment primarily as our workplace rather than someone's home, it is easy to ignore such boundaries. In addition to the routine encroachment on a person's bedroom, many other workers pass through the common living areas to get from one location to another, increasing both the commotion of the environment and the sense of strangers constantly coming and going, unconnected to the people who live there.

With regard to dignity and respect, this lack of recognition of the sanctity of one's home often results in a multitude of other negative interactions. While these are too numerous to list, a few prominent examples include failing to preserve modesty during personal care, discussing a person's challenges in public areas, or creating excessive noise and commotion while working.

As I noted at the end of the last chapter, the critical need for connectedness in our lives does not invalidate the importance of privacy. Connectedness and privacy are both experiences we choose at certain times, and the environment must be equipped to offer either, when desired. There are individual variations regarding when a person prefers solitude, but certain activities, such as sleeping, dressing, bathing, and toilet use, should be afforded absolute privacy, or else one will never feel totally secure.

Challenges of Physical Safety

"Is it safe?" For those of a certain age, this line will forever be associated with a particularly harrowing scene from John Schlesinger's 1976

film *Marathon Man*. In that scene, Sir Laurence Olivier (playing a Nazi war criminal), tortures Dustin Hoffman with a dentist's drill. Between episodes of inflicted pain, Olivier repeatedly asks if "it" is safe, Hoffman has no idea what he has stumbled into, and the popularity of dentists hit an all-time low.

The irony of the scene for me was the constant questioning about safety in the midst of an interaction that was anything but safe. Can I tie all of this into the care of people living with dementia? *Mais bien sûr!*

For many of the stakeholders involved in elder care, "security" means keeping the person physically safe at all costs. So we focus our efforts on preventing falls or unobserved "elopement" from home or nursing home. Are these risks real? Certainly. But what is the risk of only focusing on one aspect of security? Can it actually make people feel *less* secure?

From the standpoint of maintaining safety from physical harm, many of the decisions made by long-term care organizations and families alike come from a "worst-case scenario" mentality that seeks to minimize risk, but may have the opposite effect. A perfect example of this is the use of physical restraints and alarms.

Physical restraints were used for decades in an attempt to prevent falls. Little attention was paid to the indignity and emotional harm of such devices because the desire to avoid injury (and liability) was paramount. Restraints have now been largely eliminated, due to a combination of efforts on the humanitarian and elder rights fronts, as well as a body of emerging research that showed that fall prevention was minimal and was overshadowed by the health risks of restraints. (In fact, studies have shown an *increase* in serious injuries among physically restrained individuals due to factors such as heightened anxiety and discomfort from being tied, coupled with muscle weakness and deconditioning from immobilization.)

Bed and chair alarms were instituted as an aid to removing restraints while monitoring the attempts of people to stand and walk. Time has now shown these to be equally problematic, for many reasons. First, even though alarms (like restraints) intuitively seem to be a good way to prevent falls, the research has not borne this out. Often, an alarm merely alerts people to the fact that someone has already fallen, and the number of instances when a care partner can actually intervene to prevent an impending fall are few.

A second drawback, nicely explained in presentations by consultants Cathie Brady and Barbara Frank (2010), is that the use of alarms discourages critical thinking skills. In the Prologue, I use a cough/pneumonia metaphor to show that distress is often mistakenly seen as the problem, rather than a symptom of a larger need. In a similar way, an alarm being triggered is often seen as the problem; as a result, staff will all too often simply respond in such a way as to make the noise stop. They will tell the person to "sit down," and help her back into the chair or bed, sometimes several times an hour, without taking time to consider the underlying reason why the person is trying to get up.

A third and very significant problem is the sound of the alarm itself. Once again, this reflects how our "solutions" are so often centered in our own reality and operational needs, instead of trying to understand the experience of the person. Think back for a moment to our childhood years, the time of life that is so durable in the memories of the forgetful. What did our early childhood schooling tell us that an alarm meant? It meant "danger"; it meant "get out of here to a safe location."

So if a person stands up or shifts her weight such that a loud alarm sounds, what would she be expected to think—that she should calmly sit back down? Not likely. So with a bit of insight, it becomes immediately obvious that alarms would *increase* both anxiety and the urge to get up and go, not decrease them. In fact, a qualitative assessment of falls conducted by the Empira Collaborative Facilities in Minnesota in their member homes found that the sudden loud noises in the person's environment were among the most common causes of those falls (Guildermann, S. A., Jaeger, M., & Morris, C., 2013). Two common sources of these noises were loud comments by care staff and the alarms themselves. It should come as no surprise, then, that many homes that have eliminated the use of such alarms have seen a *decrease* in falls as a result.

Segregated Living and Security

Many, if not most, long-term care communities have some people with dementia living in integrated environments in addition to those living in their segregated areas. How do they decide who lives where? Often it comes down to safety concerns. In many cases, the major difference between the segregated and integrated living areas is that the former environment is locked, to prevent an unwanted exit by its residents.

More often than not, it is the primary reason for moving a person to such an environment. This is a common feature of the segregated community, stemming from an assessment of potential risk for injury due to leaving the premises, and a "one-size-fits-all" solution of locking and/ or alarming the doors. In most cases, this succeeds in keeping people inside; but just as we saw with restraints and alarms, does it truly provide security?

Once again, this is a practice that discourages critical-thinking skills. People do not attempt to leave an area simply because they have dementia; there usually is a need or desire driving the attempt. (I like to think of it as representing either a need to find something that is not available there, or to get away from something that is there.) But the use of a lock and alarm takes away our impetus to try to understand what that need or desire might be; we simply lock the door and return to our tasks, knowing that people will not get outside.

Imagine that the person feels a need to leave because of one of a variety of concerns—that her children may need attention, that he has to go home from work, that she needs some exercise and fresh air, or simply that this place just does not feel like a place where he wants to stay all day. What will the reaction of each of these individuals be when confronted by a locked door? "You cannot go to your children," "You cannot leave work," "You cannot get any fresh air," or "You must stay in this place that you do not like."

So once again, we have a staff-centered solution that actually *decreases* the person's sense of security and *increases* both the level of anxiety and the very desire to leave as well! The person returns repeatedly to the locked door, bangs on the door, calls out for help, or otherwise expresses her distress. It is another self-fulfilling prophecy, as the "special care unit" proves to be the home of the "most agitated residents."

A few years ago, I gave a series of talks at Laguna Honda Hospital and Rehab in San Francisco. They have since moved to a bright new complex next door, but at that time people were still living and working in a very old building with many antiquated structural elements.

During my tour, I was shown a locked ward for 28 men with moderate to severe dementia. The challenges of this old physical design were many—28 people were housed with 14 beds lined up along one wall and 14 more along the other, with bookshelf-style dividers added after every few beds to try to reduce the feeling of a large crowded space.

A lot of agitation occurred during the day, with occasional physical altercations as well. Oliva Ignacio, the nurse manager who led my visit, told me that she had been working to try to convince her staff that medications were not the solution to people's distress, but many remained unconvinced.

A few moments later, Oliva mentioned that there were occasional "outings" for the men. I asked her how many people they took on an outing, and she replied, "All of them, as long as no one is sick. We have a big bus we use." I asked her how many staff attended to them on these outings and was told that the usual complement accompanied, plus an activity professional. I asked how often altercations occurred during these outings and she said, "Never."

"There's your argument," I responded. I suggested that the care team discuss the reasons why the men would be so distressed inside the living environment, and yet so much better off when they went on outings. In this case, both the crowding and the locked door were contributing to what was almost certainly a claustrophobic and intrusive situation for these men. In other words, this secure ward offered little security.

Another telling story from this ward was of a gentleman who became quite agitated on a regular basis. He was quite calm and pleasant when taken for a walk outside the ward, but upon returning and seeing the locked doors, he invariably stopped and would not go back inside. There was only one nursing assistant who had a special knack for convincing him to go back inside.

At that time, the solution of the staff had been to only take him for walks when that particular staff member was working; as a result, there were many days or shifts when his need was not being met. One of my discussions with staff that day revolved around setting up a team meeting whereby the nursing assistant could share her wisdom and insights with her fellow care partners, so that others could also develop "the knack" that she had.

Organizations will often adopt other, less-restrictive approaches to prevent unwanted egress, in addition to or instead of locked doors. Examples include murals painted on doors and elevators, dark floor patterns in front of doors or elevators that stop people with visuospatial difficulties, stop signs, or doors that lead into circular hallways or courtyards but do not lead off of the campus.

Once again, these may provide an effective means to keep people from leaving, but do they increase their sense of security? How often does a painting of a meadow on a door or elevator confuse someone or give him the impression that he can easily step outside? How often do people become stressed when there appears to be a hole in the floor in front of the elevator? How often do people view such barriers as challenges that actually hold their attention and increase their desire to get past them? And how often do these tactics lull us into a false sense of security that blinds us to the real needs that underlie such "elopement behaviors?"

Another barrier to security that arises from segregated living is the anxiety that can result from having a higher concentration of people in one's environment who may be confused, distressed, or likewise not able to respect personal boundaries. (Keep in mind, however, that in most long-term care environments the largest group of "intrusive wanderers" is the professional staff!)

A final barrier to mention here arises from the common stigmas surrounding dementia discussed in Chapter 3. If care partners succumb to the notion that people are "no longer there," then there will be less attention to the basics of privacy, dignity, and respect in day-to-day conversation and care. Shanks (1999) expresses the potential danger of a view that sees the person as less than whole:

> There is no element more central or more necessary to excellent careproviding than the acceptance of the [Alzheimer's] patient as a human being, yet this basic concept of the humanness of the patient is all too often overlooked. When we deny another's humanness, however, we deny the existence of that person's inner spirit or soul. One reason slavery endured for so long in America was that some proponents promoted the idea that the Africans had no souls. It is a dangerous and degenerate society that engages in the dehumanization of any segment of its population.
>   . . . Yet being human includes both sickness and wellness, good and evil, old and new, positive and negative, saint and sinner. (p. 31)

While the potential for a less-than-whole view of people living with dementia can occur in all environments, do not assume that "special care units" are immune to this type of thinking. While there are some very enlightened organizations out there, many more have segregated people based on an operational model that is very much rooted in the traditional biomedical view, complete with all of its assumptions and stigmas. The term *special care unit* nearly always implies a locked door, but it does not necessarily mean "special care" of the person-centered variety.

Community-Based Living and Security

Most of the challenges to security mentioned in earlier sections apply to community-based living as well, from unfamiliar home care workers to immodest personal care to stigmatizing words and negative body language. But there are a few others that deserve mention. The familiarity of one's home and family members would be expected to better support one's sense of security compared to an unfamiliar nursing home, but some aspects of community living can erode security as well.

When the Familiar Becomes Unfamiliar

As we discussed with identity, the home environment may be rock-stable, but one's brain is evolving and processing input from this environment differently over time. Without attention to this, the familiar can become unfamiliar, and the trusted untrustworthy in the face of short-term memory loss. As Shouse (2006) explained,

> These days, Mom's life is like a trust-building exercise, where you bond with a group of strangers, then fall backwards into their waiting arms. For Mom, most everyone is now a stranger, and most every event, from eating to getting into the car to walking into this house, demands trust. (p. 83)

Many people living at home have milder cognitive disability and are acutely aware of, and compensating for, their changing experiences. Once again, the brain is not in a pure state of decay—it is actively engaged in problem solving and creating compensatory mechanisms for what has been lost. Part of that involves the establishment of routines that help keep the person grounded in a world where memories are ever changing.

Rose (2003) relates the story of meeting his friend, Pam, at her office. He had limited his driving to familiar places such as this, and he decided to carpool with her to a nearby coffee shop for lunch. But as he engaged in conversation with her, problems developed as they drove:

> I wasn't paying any attention to where she was going when she left the parking lot. I was talking when I should have been watching where we were going. It is very important to me that I know exactly where I am at every moment. If I have the feeling of being lost, I start to panic. She was taking a different route than I do, and suddenly I was in strange surroundings. I could hardly take it.
> "Stop, Pam, you are going to have to go back to the parking lot."
> "Did you forget something?"
> "No. I am lost."
> "Oh, don't worry, I am going to bring you back," she said.
> "No! You don't understand, I don't know where I am. I must
> go back to my truck to get straightened out." (She slowed to turn

around when I recognized the fire station.) "I know where I am now, Pam, it's okay."

The damage was done. When I panic like that, I don't do anything right for a time. I can't talk, or walk. It is like this thing is my head [*sic*] is spinning out of control. (p. 6)

Shanks (1999) describes walks around the neighborhood with her husband. On these occasions, she became aware that he had retained old habits and superstitions as a way of feeling secure, and his longstanding caring nature kept him acutely aware of the potential for others to be in peril:

On our walks, he still jumps over mud puddles and steps around cracks in the sidewalk. If there is an obstruction in our path, he presses my hand to steer me away from what he perceives as danger. Two or three years ago, if we saw a small child alone on the street as we walked by, he would become very agitated, slowing down and looking back, pointing to the child. I am sure he thought the child was lost. Each time I had to reassure him that everything was all right before he would continue on our walk. (p. 35)

Inner Struggles of the Changing Mind

Camp (2012) also reminds us that as people become increasingly forgetful, some of their "denial" may be an ego defense mechanism. The fact of living with a condition such as Alzheimer's threatens one's security by challenging one's sense of self. This helps explain the reactions of some people, particularly those who are in an early phase of the illness, when deficits (such as repetitive questioning) are pointed out to them. Camp explains that being told that you have asked the same question three times when you did not recall doing so creates an internal conflict:

Now you must make a hard decision. Is your friend lying or telling the truth? If you believe your friend is lying, then you are going to drive home with a person you cannot trust. . . . On the other hand, if your friend is telling the truth, then there is something wrong with you. (p. 6)

So any situation that shakes confidence and instills doubt can threaten security. For this reason, many people living in the community become increasingly isolated in their homes, due to social experiences during which a person's comments or actions caused a reaction in others that challenged their sense of security, or brought embarrassment to them or their family. But decreasing social connections has its own risks; being confined to one space, and increasingly alone with one's thoughts, can also threaten security. This is often the genesis of the restlessness that people display when no simple cause is evident:

> Many people have tried to guess why Alzheimer's disease patients are so restless and want to walk around at all hours of the day and night. I believe I may have a clue. When the darkness and emptiness fill my mind, it is totally terrifying. I cannot think my way out of it. It stays there, and sometimes images stay stuck in my mind. Thoughts increasingly haunt me. The only way that I can break this cycle is to move. Vigorous exercise to the point of exhaustion gets my mind out of the black hole. . . . Now I try to schedule my daily routine with productive, physically demanding activity. Following this, I rest quietly, listening to my tapes and sometimes fall asleep. When I awake, I am refreshed and usually more alert mentally. (Davis, 1989, p. 96)

Intrusions of the Past

With the process of dementia, there is often a shifting of the person's focus toward other parts of her life. These may be events that happened long ago and are more deeply ingrained in her memory; they may also be events that carry a strong emotional connection. The focus on events that may have been stressful in the past creates another challenge to security. In many cases, unresolved trauma can reawaken, causing a type of posttraumatic stress disorder.

Many older people have experienced war, illness and death of loved ones, poverty, or physical or sexual abuse. Once again, getting to know the person's history is often critical to finding clues to distress. Camp (2012) relates one such story:

> A woman in an assisted living facility who had early-stage dementia was coming to the nurses' station on a regular basis and asking the question, "Is it safe here?" They would tell her that it was, and then later she would repeat the process. This would happen many, many, many times throughout the day and evening . . .
>
> . . . It turned out that she had been living alone in an apartment for independent seniors before moving into the assisted living residence. When she lived in the senior apartment, a burglar had entered while she was there, robbed her, and beaten her up. She had a good reason to worry about her safety. To address her need, the nurses put a large sign at the nurses' station that said, "You are safe here." When the

older woman would approach the station, staff would simply point at the sign, which she could read from many feet away. The resident would smile and go back to what she had been doing. With repetition, staff did not even have to point at the sign. The woman would look at it whenever she felt the need for reassurance about her safety. (pp. 52–53)

Many care partners report seeing episodes of distress among war veterans when an alarm, an intercom, a televised image, or even a general level of commotion in the vicinity triggers memories of a battle. Holocaust survivors and other former prisoners of war are particularly sensitive to such trappings as institutional showers or feelings of being controlled by others.

Lastly, changes in mental maps of familiar places, and in procedural memory, may cause people to have difficulty navigating, even within the confines of their own home. Shanks (1999) closed off sections of her house in order to reduce the available space her husband needed to remember how to navigate. By creating some boundaries, she was able to provide both a sense of security and also autonomy, as he became more empowered to use his living space successfully.

Accommodations to Physical Space

You might ask, how does limiting accessible space as Shanks did differ from a locked or alarmed unit? An important factor is whether the domains of well-being are fulfilled within the space. For many in locked units, the desire to leave reflects a lack of fulfillment of well-being within the living space. When that need is fulfilled, the desire is often eliminated.

In 2012, St. John's Home in Rochester, New York, opened the first two Green House® homes in the nation to be moved off of a campus for older adults and integrated into a diverse residential community. Initially, a few of the people who moved in became restless and would try to leave. Although the doors of the house had an exit alarm, the staff recognized that a certain amount of disorientation was likely to accompany any move, even to lovely houses such as these. There was no familiarity with the homes and the elders were still not well known to their care partners.

What happened over time was that the houses became more of a "fit" for those elders, as the staff recognized their individual personalities and preferences and began to create more meaningful daily interactions. As the care partners, the physical environment, and the daily rhythms of life became more familiar, and in the absence of institutional trappings that would have made the homes feel foreign, even those living with severe cognitive limitations became more secure in their surroundings, and more trusting of the dedicated, caring staff. The staff also became more aware of what triggered people's restlessness, and began to preemptively engage them or take them for walks when these signs occurred.

After several weeks a team meeting was held, because people walking too close to the doors were triggering the exit alarms and disturbing the tranquility of the houses. On further discussion, it was noted that no one was actually trying to leave anymore—they were simply passing within range of the sensors and their wander-alert bracelets were triggering the alarms. At this point, the staff also had to take on a level of trust—trust that they now knew their elders well enough to understand their rhythms, and that they had created a better sense of familiarity and security in the homes among those living with dementia. Taking a collective deep breath, the staff decided to remove the alarm bracelets, and the residents continue to relax in their homes without further attempts to leave.

At times, the identity or purpose of a room or object becomes misinterpreted and sometimes the best answer is to create other boundaries to help the person be more successful. Shanks (1999) found that extinguishing a light in an adjoining room helped decrease her husband's need to get up and explore at night—the light was triggering a sense of insecurity that needed to be investigated. Her solution was to "guide" him to bed at night by turning off the living room lights and turning on the light beside his bed, which drew him to that room.

She also found that he was using a walk-in closet in the bedroom to urinate, apparently mistaking it for the bathroom. Nailing the closet door shut led him to redraw his mental map to a proper alignment. Shanks equated this to other modifications people make for physical disabilities:

> I have been asked how I could just nail a closet shut. My answer is, how could I not nail his closet shut? How could the use of a closet compare to doing what is necessary to keep Hughes in his own home? Our daughter-in-law, Chris, observed that when a family member has a physical illness, we think nothing of making the structural changes necessary to facilitate home care. But not so with family members who have what we call mental illnesses (as if mental illnesses have no connection to the body). Nothing material compares to the value of a human life. (p. 47)

The Special Problems of "All-or-None Thinking" and "Surplus Safety"

When it comes to security (and autonomy as well), there are two common practices that create significant problems in all living environments. One practice, *all-or-none thinking*, reflects a view that is polarized and does not accommodate individual nuances. The other, *surplus safety*, involves seeing only one aspect of a two-sided coin. Both of these practices arise from a combination of stigmas regarding dementia, preconceived notions of the ability of the person to participate in life choices, and inability to be flexible or to individualize care (either because of the institutional priorities of long-term care environments, or because of inadequate support in community-based living). These practices create many of our toughest challenges in caring for people living with cognitive changes.

All-or-none thinking leads us to make decisions based on a limited view of options, and often falls short of enhancing well-being. An example is the common dilemma faced by care partners in all environments regarding how to answer a comment or question that is not grounded in our reality. I am often asked to help people choose between the two extremes of telling the bald truth (risking further emotional upset) or using a "little white lie" to calm or distract the person.

When faced with this simple either/or choice, most people opt for the white lie, which seems less harmful in the long run. The problem with this is that our fabrication does not fulfill the need behind the question, and therefore the doubt and insecurity will remain. Furthermore, it assumes that the person will swallow the line and not remember if our invented scenario (e.g., "Your children are being picked up from school and will be over in an hour") does not come to pass. But all too often when we weave such a tangled web, the person will recognize when our answer does not prove to be true. The result is that we have eroded their trust, and therefore their sense of security.

It is human nature to long for black-and-white choices in order to simplify the many situations we encounter. But this type of thinking creates a trap—for us as well as the person with dementia. As we will see in Chapter 7, there is a third option in this scenario that leads to a more durable solution.

All-or-none thinking also underlies many of the interactions described that erode privacy, dignity, and respect. If the person is not fully cognitively able, we too often assume that the basic underpinnings of dignified interaction are no longer necessary.

The other common form of all-or-none thinking surrounds issues of autonomy and empowerment: Dad can drive a car until he cannot, and then we take the keys away; Mom can live alone until she cannot, and then we force her to move; if Dad can no longer remember the date, then he cannot make choices about life-sustaining treatment; if Mom does not remember her daughter's name, the staff will choose her meals for her.

There are multiple levels of empowerment that will be discussed thoroughly in the next chapter. I mention these examples here to show how this type of thinking leads to our second practice: surplus safety.

Surplus safety has been brought to the level of discussion and debate to a great extent through the efforts of Drs. Bill Thomas and Judah Ronch. Here is the basic premise:

> In discussions revolving around daily life and care, safety is an area of high concern. Family members, nursing home regulators, and liability insurers alike focus intently on the process of minimizing risk. But the focus of these discussions only sees one face of the "two-sided risk coin."
>
> Traditional risk discussions focus on *downside risk*—the risk that an event will turn out worse than expected. If a person goes outside, what are the chances he will get lost, or walk into traffic? If he walks unassisted, what are the chances he will fall and be injured? If she goes to a social event, what are the chances she will be overwhelmed and distressed by the environment. When seen purely from this angle, minimizing risk seems reasonable.
>
> But there is another side to the coin, which can be called *upside risk*—the risk that an event will turn out better than expected. Reconsider the above scenarios: If a person goes outside, what are the chances he will improve his conditioning and overall mood and sleep better at night? If he walks unassisted, could it improve his balance and even lead to greater independence with other activities of daily living? If she goes to a social event, could it bring meaning and growth to her as a person and forestall further cognitive decline?
>
> Viewed from this angle, simply minimizing downside risk can stifle well-being. Indeed, there is often a connection: Reducing the chance of any bad outcome also reduces the chance of any good outcome. So safety and quality of life are often perched on a seesaw—when one goes up, the other goes down.

> Surplus safety arises when we only seek to minimize downside risk without consideration of potential benefits. It is driven by a combination of a societal mentality of avoiding liability at all costs, plus the all-or-none thinking that blinds us to seeing that intermediate solutions exist that can manage risk within reasonable parameters, without leading to irresponsible decisions.

As a lead-in to the next section on enhancing security, I suggest another response to the surplus safety scenario. A better approach should seek a plan that, rather than minimizing risk, *negotiates* risk.

The essence of the concept of negotiated risk is that all of life involves a degree of risk-taking. Every time we get into a car, board a train or airplane, or open our mouths to speak our minds we are taking one sort of risk or another. But we accept these risks with the knowledge that they enable us to continue to engage with the world, and with the expectation that our actions will lead to new experiences that create meaning, growth, and joy in our lives.

We take many of these risks without even thinking of them, because the potential benefit is so much greater that there is no need to consider not going forward. Yet the diagnosis of dementia causes us to scrutinize risk in microscopic detail, and to magnify the downside, while failing to realize the upside potential. We must disabuse ourselves of the notion that we can ever eliminate risk from anyone's life. As Thomas (2012) once stated, "The only risk-free human environment is a coffin."

Negotiating risk is neither the elimination of any activity that might produce a downside, nor the acceptance of all activities without boundaries. It is a conversation about who the person is, how he stands to benefit from engaging in an activity, what the downside risks are and if they can be mitigated to an acceptable degree with the support of the person's care partners. This process requires identity and connectedness— one cannot make such a determination without knowing the individual, involving the individual in the conversation to the greatest extent that he is able, and creating a network of support for the individual in his efforts.

An example of negotiated risk might involve driving a car. Many people living with dementia clearly are not capable of driving. But many who have had some difficulties with certain aspects of driving might be able to continue to a limited extent under the right circumstances. For example, if reaction speed is slowed due to age or illness, then driving may be limited to certain speeds and certain roads. Other guidelines might involve driving only within a limited area, driving only in the daytime or in good weather, or perhaps driving with a family member accompanying. Such decisions should be reevaluated and revisited periodically to be sure that the benefit continues to justify the risk.

I realize that I have chosen a "hot button item" for my example. Many readers may feel that there is no justification for a person with a diagnosis of dementia to drive under any circumstances—the potential liability is just too great. I believe that with careful planning, we do not always have to go to one extreme or the other. The main reason for using this scenario is to demonstrate that if something as challenging as driving can be discussed with respect to negotiating risk, then there are a multitude of smaller decisions that also deserve these efforts, in order to enhance both security and autonomy. There will be much more discussion of other aspects of empowerment in Chapter 6.

Enhancing Security

In the face of such a daunting array of challenges, it may seem overwhelming to try to make inroads into improving a person's security. However, there is much that can be done to address both the intrinsic and extrinsic challenges to this important domain of well-being. This is a critical juncture, and care partners need to devote much effort to this domain if higher aspects of well-being are ever to be realized.

In addressing the challenges listed earlier, we will start with two important philosophical points. First, each challenge already listed has antidotes that can be provided through personal, operational, and physical transformation of the living environment. Second, the larger areas of risk that may seem insurmountable are very much a symptom of lack of security in smaller areas. When careful attention is paid to providing security in these smaller areas, many of the larger concerns will disappear.

Consider the example of attempts to leave a nursing home. This may often reflect a lack of security in the many smaller interactions and events the person experiences throughout the day. When these are properly attended to, the larger desire to leave the building often goes away because the person feels more secure.

That is why it is always best to start by addressing the "little things." They are easier to visualize, the results are more easily attained, and the cumulative effect on the person makes the larger issues easier to address. Starting small also means less downside risk in the early going, and the learning curve helps make the larger risks easier to negotiate down the road.

A parallel philosophy is seen in the old financial adage, "If you watch your nickels and dimes, the dollars will take care of themselves." Start with baby steps. And as we will discuss in the next chapter, this same philosophy will be a key to enhancing autonomy through progressive empowerment steps.

Personal Transformation

We begin where the discussion of challenges started: with the loss of familiarity and trust. While a large part of this is due to intrinsic changes in the brain, there is much we can do to restore familiarity and trust, even for those who are very forgetful. For our first steps, recall that security arises from our first two domains: identity and connectedness.

Identity involves deep knowing; for familiarity and trust, this needs to flow in both directions. It is important for the care partner to know the person well; this knowledge will guide the best approaches to interaction and conversation, help one understand what situations threaten the person's feelings of security, and help one know how best to allay the person's fears. When language is challenged, this deep knowing also helps the care partner to understand the difficulties that the person may not be able to express in words.

But it is also important for the person living with dementia to develop familiarity with the care partners. This is the foundation of trust. Even if you do not know where you might be headed, it is easier to place your trust in a friend than in a stranger. When the care partners share details of their own personal lives, it broadens the person's knowledge of who they are beyond the tasks they perform. Seeing care partners as whole people can also ease the person's sense of anxiety, especially during personal care.

This two-way familiarity enhances connectedness, which is so important for those with short-term memory problems. Even though the details of the person's physical environment and events of the day may be hard to recall, a familiar face can make the surroundings feel safer, even when the person feels physically displaced from home. (A parallel in our own lives is that it is far easier to attend a social gathering in an unfamiliar place if there are friends attending as well.)

In order to build familiarity, it is also important to embrace the belief that people with dementia can learn new information. There may be more repetition required, but new memories do form, particularly when information is presented consistently from consistent sources. And where security is concerned, the emotional memory of a familiar person is more important in creating trust than remembering all the details of names and dates.

Therefore, from an interpersonal standpoint, it is also paramount that care partners use all of the "face-to-face" communication skills described in Chapter 9 of *Dementia Beyond Drugs* (Power, 2010) in every interaction in order to optimize their connection to the person. Careful attention to body language and the skill of "being present" during conversation is critical to presenting oneself in a manner that will build trust.

Many people underestimate just how much can be done to help an anxious person feel secure, simply by sharing a calm presence. One's own sense of calm can act as a life raft for someone swimming in uncertainty. In fact, using our body language to promote calm is often necessary before any calming words can be processed and understood. (For a real-life example, see *Dementia Beyond Drugs*, pp. 155–157.)

In *Out of Solitude: Three Meditations of the Christian Life* (2004), Henri J. M. Nouwen notes:

> The friend who can be silent with us in a moment of despair or confusion, who can stay with us in an hour of grief and bereavement, who can tolerate not knowing, not curing, not healing and face with us the reality of our powerlessness, that is the friend who cares. (p. 38)

When the time comes for a verbal response, Tena Alonzo (2013) from Beatitudes in Phoenix, Arizona, suggests we consider the following: "That sounds really scary. I will keep you safe." This follows the guideline from Chapter 4 of validating the emotion expressed first, to ensure the best connection with the person in her present reality.

Finally, the language we use in everyday discourse must paint the person and her actions in a manner that is humane, nonjudgmental, and nonstigmatized, so that we (and others around us) do not unconsciously adopt body language that defeats our attempts to provide care and support. Nolan's Senses framework (2006) maintains that security involves protecting one's innate worth and rights as a human being, regardless of diagnosis.

Earlier, I promised to share a simple guideline for choosing language that helps us move to a more positive view of the person in need. Next time you are engaged in discussing a situation regarding a person living with dementia, follow this simple rule: *Do not use any words that you would not want used to describe you, or someone you love.* Would you like to be called a "behavior problem?" If not, drop it. Would you feel uncomfortable being labeled "difficult," "nasty," "belligerent," or "acting out?" Likewise.

Try the above exercise in your next team meeting. It is amazing how quickly people become tongue-tied when they cannot use such labeling language—such is the extent to which these words have become ingrained in our culture. But security (and indeed humanity) begins and ends right here.

Improving our language is a continuous process and needs to be revisited periodically. In *Dementia Beyond Drugs*, I used the term *physical aggression*. Since that time, I have challenged my own language, as the term implies a desire to injure others, rather than a response to being put in a difficult position. Since I would not wish to be labeled "aggressive," I no longer use the term to describe others.

It is important to reemphasize that our focus on language must also extend to our written communications. If anything, the medical chart creates even more powerful images and associations in our minds than the spoken word because it is an official document. And once a word or phrase is used, there is a tendency for others to co-opt the same language in their future documentations:

> I was doing an expert review of a medical record for an attorney whose law firm was defending a nursing home against a liability suit. In this case, a woman living with dementia had been on an antipsychotic drug for nearly 3 years, and I was concerned about any possible contribution of the drug to her medical problems and eventual death.
>
> Starting with the last entry, I began tracing the use of the drug through the chart in reverse, to find the starting date and reason for its use. The last medical entry stated that she was "an 89-year-old woman with a history of dementia and hallucinations." Each previous medical note started with the same notation, yet no description was given as to what type of "hallucinations" she might have had. After several entries, I reached a point where she became "an 88-year-old woman with a history of dementia and hallucinations," and 12 months farther back, "an 87-year-old . . ." However, nowhere in the

doctors' or nurses' notes was there a record of anything that justified the diagnosis.

Finally, over 2 years before the final entry, I found a single nurse's note that described a comment the woman had made that sounded confused, but was more likely a misinterpretation of the environment than a true hallucination. But the label "hallucinations" was put in writing and simply copied over from month to month, year to year, without question, even though no other events ever occurred. And the drug was continued the entire time as well.

At one of my seminars I was asked if it was not okay to use potentially stigmatizing language in the medical record, given that much of that terminology was endemic in the profession and used commonly in medical and nursing education. My response was (and is) that our medical language needs to evolve just as medical care does. We no longer use once-common terms such as *idiocy* (for congenital hypothyroidism) or *mongolism* (for Down syndrome), because we have come to see that such terms are offensive. The same fate should befall any terms that dehumanize the person living with cognitive illness.

Furthermore, as previously described, language can affect our own body language and demeanor, rendering our care less effective and potentially worsening distress. Any terminology that has the potential to negatively impact well-being and care is not up to professional standards of care.

At this juncture, I will acknowledge that there is also a movement afoot to remove the word *dementia* from the lexicon. The word comes from the Latin root meaning insane ("out of mind"). Many people feel that the stigmas surrounding this family of conditions are such that the word must be eliminated in order for us to truly get past them. In fact, the authors of the new *Diagnostic and Statistical Manual of Mental Disorders*, fifth edition (DSM-5) have proposed dropping the word in favor of two classifications: "minor or major neurocognitive disorders."

I will not explore here all of the ramifications of this change, but I wrote an extensive blog essay on the topic shortly after the proposed change was publicized (Power, 2012b). Psychologist Dr. Nader Shabahangi uses the term *forgetfulness*, which he finds much less stigmatizing. He acknowledges that the condition comprises more than simple memory loss, but finds that this is a good philosophical foundation for the evolving reality of the person in question. In a written response to my blog essay, he expressed these ideas:

The timing of your comments is quite astounding. Just yesterday I was at a "dementia" conference and less than an hour into it I had to leave; the continual use of the word "dementia," coupled with words such as "epidemic" and "crisis," was too painful to me. See, when I think of our elders who are forgetful—and to me forgetful also refers to forgetting some of our consensus behaviors and language use, not just memory loss—I think of names: Mary, Nick, David, Nancy, Tom, Bill. I think of how funny they are, how they make me slow down, how they push me to remember to smile, not to take life so seriously, to investigate more fully the question of Who I am. Yes, (Michel) Foucault and Richard (Taylor) and Al and others are right: There exists a refusal of a scientific or administrative inquisition of asking such a question with all the depth and humanity it demands to be asked.

You see, forgetfulness is a gift and there is a cure for it: I change the way I look at people who are forgetful, including myself. We live in a perceiver-dependent world where I create the world in which I live, where I "see" what I have been taught, inculcated, really, to "see" in a way that is reductionistic, that looks for shorthand labels rather than descriptions. I am part of this system myself, I do it myself. (Power, 2012b, comments section)

For the purposes of this book, I have continued to use the term *dementia* as a bridge for readers who are most familiar with the term for this family of conditions. However, I have been slowly introducing other terms, such as *forgetfulness*, to help expand our thinking on the topic. I also use *changing cognitive ability* as a tool to help us embrace the potential of seeing dementia as a different ability and the greater potential that it holds than that of a *terminal disease*. Also note that I consistently refer to the "condition" or the "illness" rather than the "disease," because of the way the latter reinforces reductionistic thinking.

Clearly, this is another area in which everyone's language, including mine, will continue to evolve. Stay tuned.

Enhancing Privacy, Dignity, and Respect

From the standpoint of privacy, dignity, and respect, there is much in the interpersonal arena to be addressed. Always knocking and asking permission before entering a room, using a preferred term of address, getting at or below eye level, and all of the other "face-to-face" specifics listed in *Dementia Beyond Drugs* set the stage for encounters that will help enhance security. Preserving modesty during personal care and avoiding potentially disparaging comments (or *any* comments about a person's needs) in public areas will enhance privacy and dignity.

There are many other details of personal interaction and care that have been discussed in *Dementia Beyond Drugs* that will not be repeated here. This is not meant to understate their importance, however. One other aspect, that of explaining each step of personal care to prepare the person for what is about to transpire, is also a powerful security enhancer and will be addressed further in the next chapter.

Operational Transformation

At the risk of being redundant, if familiarity and trust are paramount to a sense of security, then there is no better way to accomplish this than with dedicated staff assignments. What good can come from constantly challenging someone whose memory is already challenged with the additional task of reforming relationships over and over?

But taking a lesson from the previous section, it is not enough simply to see the same faces every day; careful attention to the interpersonal dynamic of those interactions must be consistent for all of those dedicated care partners. With regard to security, there is no other well-being domain in which one care partner can so drastically undo the good work of all others through negative interactions.

In fact, it is hard to overemphasize the importance of the small interpersonal encounters—verbal and nonverbal language, actions, and interactions—especially as they relate to security. If we had a pill that we knew would increase people's comfort and well-being, we would rush to use it; if a pill were found to be harmful to people, we would take pains to avoid it. We should be no less diligent with our daily interactions!

Spontaneity versus Routine

Another issue to address as a bridge from interpersonal to operational approaches is the challenging question of how we balance predictable routine versus spontaneity and variety. Variety and spontaneity are powerful antidotes to soul-crushing boredom in institutional living. But if familiarity and trust are essential to creating security, how do we weave the element of spontaneity into daily life without increasing distress?

I have been asked this question several times, and, once again, helpful guidance lies within the well-being framework, specifically here in the domain of security. We begin by avoiding an all-or-none approach and realize that both routine and spontaneity can have a place in the life of a person living with cognitive disability. The trick lies in knowing when each one works best.

An examination of this well-being domain tells us that spontaneity is likely to work best when a person's sense of security is strong, whereas predictable routine is important in situations where a person might be feeling less secure. So, for example, the time when someone is undressed and being helped with a shower is probably not the time to introduce the element of surprise, especially if the person has exhibited discomfort during this activity in the past. (This is a primary reason why the appearance of an unfamiliar care partner to help with such an intimate task usually creates distress—it introduces the element of surprise at exactly the wrong time.)

On the other hand, when feelings of security and comfort are high (such as when a person is relaxing in her room or sitting in a lounge with friends or family), then a spontaneous event (bursting into song, cracking jokes, or the sight of children or pets running into the room) would be more likely to create moments of joy and pleasure.

Removing Alarms

Operational transformation is as important as structural changes when it comes to removing alarms and decreasing the risk of someone exiting a building unsafely. The first and most important step is to reintroduce skills and processes for critical thinking to the care partner team. Repeated attempts to stand, walk, explore, or exit should trigger discussions that look at these as goal-driven actions, rather than disease-driven ones.

Long-term care organizations should take advantage of tools such as impromptu huddles, learning circles, and my Experiential Pathway to Well-Being approach (described in Chapter 10) to engage each team member and tap into everyone's knowledge of the person. Careful attention should be paid to the rhythm of the individual, as this often drives certain actions and makes them more understandable and predictable than they might initially appear.

The next step is to craft the ideal solution to fit the individual's rhythms and needs and then flex the operations to best meet those needs. It may seem daunting to create such flexibility, especially in a living area where several individuals may be using alarms or walking around freely. Can it be done?

The secret is to take small steps. I have heard of organizations that eliminated chair alarms one shift at a time, pausing after each step until successful. My personal preference is to look at these initiatives *one person at a time*; it's a smaller "bite" to take, and it also combats the mentality that separates shifts, bringing all care partners together to work more seamlessly toward the goal. And I recommend that you start with one of the easier challenges.

First, identify a person whose needs may be a bit more obvious and/or more easily met by operational shifts. Work on meeting that person's needs, day and night, until a measure of success has been achieved (e.g., alarm removed safely, or 80% to 90% reduction in exit-seeking actions). Then choose another individual and use what you have learned to identify and meet her needs.

Each successive person addressed will help the operations to shift incrementally, and there is a cumulative effect of these shifts on the entire environment. In addition, there will be a learning curve, such that the more challenging and difficult-to-decipher situations begin to become clearer. The exit alarm example from St. John's Green House homes given earlier is a good illustration of how this can happen.

As we move toward the last section on physical transformation, a word of caution: Although there are some definite structural elements to security, they do not exist independent of operations. A private room or an enclosed living area is of little benefit if the staff does not respect boundaries, or if dignity and respect are missing in daily interactions. The following section should challenge the reader to think not only about the physical space, but also about how the space is used.

Physical Transformation

In long-term care settings, a key to security is familiarity of physical surroundings. How can we optimize this when a person no longer lives in her own home, or may forget the details of her previous home?

First of all, the advice on size from the last chapter is relevant for security as well as connectedness. Small environments maintain a homier feel and are easier to navigate and commit to memory. They also necessarily have fewer people living and working there, as well as less potential for noise and commotion.

Familiarity also lies in the décor and trappings of the living space. Many organizations rush to create an upscale décor more akin to a modern luxury hotel. It looks good when one is taking a tour, but who among us would feel comfortable living in even a fine hotel week in, week out? Hotels are made to satisfy a common denominator of needs, and eventually we will long for a more personal space that conforms to our unique rhythms.

In chronicling his mother's journey with Alzheimer's, Wong (2009) describes her concern around the possibility of having to move out of her own apartment. She expressed her feelings this way:

> A pigsty, to a pig, is still home. My own place, my own ways. Other people's place, other people's ways. (p. 159)

Even if imperfect, a space that retains identity and connectedness will feel familiar and secure. That connectedness is also a function of the diverse daily interactions available to people within the living space. Having consulted on designs for aging populations all over the world, environmental gerontologist Dr. Emi Kiyota (2011) has reached this conclusion:

> Elders living in grass huts in Africa with children at their feet are often happier than people in assisted living homes with a chandelier over their heads.

Private Bedrooms

We have already discussed ways to bring identity and connectedness into the physical space. Another important component of security is privacy. And here we must pose another challenge to our current system of care.

Let us not beat around the bush: Our elders in long-term living environments deserve privacy, no less than any of us. This means that the place where they sleep, use the toilet, conduct sensitive conversations, and express their sexual intimacy must be completely private. The only way to accomplish this is with a private room with a closeable door.

Once again, this seemingly obvious fact flies in the face of standard practice. No doubt, financial concerns regarding square footage of living space have driven the construction of shared rooms over the years. Along with this is the pervasive ageism of the institutional model, an approach that assumes older or frail individuals no longer have a need or right to that which the rest of us take for granted.

While working at St. John's Home in Rochester, I was once stopped in the hallway by two of our veteran nurses. They pulled me aside with an earnest look and said, "Dr. Power, we believe our elders are too old to have to 'go back to college!'" Amen to that. (In fact, unlike nursing homes, at least colleges make an effort to collect a simple personality profile in an attempt to find good roommate matches.)

Even though the retrofitting of thousands of nursing homes in a slow economy may be too daunting, I strongly believe that *no new construction or renovation should be undertaken without providing private rooms and bathrooms for all*. How much money is saved with double rooms compared against the time spent by staff addressing roommate conflicts, distress due to feelings of lack of security, and the excess disability caused by living in an environment that erodes one's well-being? On top of that, the very real and increasing problem of resistant infections demands frequent moves when the affected person shares a room.

When discussing this concept with operators and architects, I start with the following as my top two arguments for private rooms for all:

1. Whenever a "VIP," such as a board member, a benefactor, or his relative, needs to spend time in our nursing home, what is the one constant? The person receives a private room. Why is that? Because this is one of the primary ways that we show the individual that we value and respect him for his contribution to our organization. Therefore, we acknowledge that privacy is a precious commodity, and providing privacy is a way of bestowing honor on those we value. But what does that say about how we view our other guests, those who do not receive this respectful gesture?

2. For those who still feel that a person in long-term care no longer needs privacy, I offer this scenario: Imagine that tonight you are home having dinner with your family. There is a knock at the door, and two men come into your house or apartment, carrying a mattress and bedspring. The men set the bed up in your bedroom across from your bed, hang a thin curtain between the two beds, and then escort a stranger into the home who will share your bedroom and bathroom for the rest of your life. How many of you are ready and willing to take on this type of living arrangement?

The truth is, even those of us who are in good health could suddenly experience a motor vehicle accident or a stroke, leading to a need for skilled care. This may not be some hypothetical situation we will face far into the future. Who among us is ready to surrender our privacy tomorrow?

The two primary arguments I have heard in favor of double rooms, particularly for people living with dementia, are (1) many of them seem to form a good relationship with their roommates, and (2) they may even obtain a sense of security by not being alone in their room at night. I refute both with two counterarguments.

First, individuals are extremely adaptable to adversity; that is how people have survived horrendous conditions throughout history. When forced to share a room with no choice in the matter, many people learn to "make the best of the situation." Through close proximity, they may well become friends with their roommates. However, friendship has its limits; many of us have close friends, but rarely do we sleep in the same room or share the same bathroom with them on a regular basis. Kiyota also reminds us that people will be less likely to socially engage if they are not afforded an optimum level of privacy in their living environment (personal communication, November 4, 2013). They will feel less secure and will spend their time seeking privacy and withdrawing, rather than engaging.

Second, if people gain feelings of security from having another person living in their room, it means that the care environment has not done enough to fulfill their sense of security. Perhaps staff members are entering without warning, or rotation of care partners results in "strangers" frequenting people's rooms. In such a case, the roommate provides the familiarity and trust that the care partners have failed to create. It is a band-aid for a broken system of care, not a preferred arrangement.

The bottom line is for each of us to ask ourselves: Should we need to move to a home tomorrow, next week, next year, would we prefer a private room or a shared room with a stranger we did not choose? It would be a rare person who would not opt for the private room. Remember, our policies and practices today create the future we may well inherit for ourselves.

One last comment about private rooms: I write this as a citizen of the United States, and although many countries are similar in their outlook, I realize that there are cultural differences in how people regard privacy. Each community should hold discussions on security and privacy, viewed through their cultural lens. But every discussion also needs to embrace the perspective of those who actually live in these environments, not just the operators and designers.

Combining Private Space with Operations

As already mentioned, operational factors contribute to privacy as well. Staff and visitors must respect the boundaries of residents' rooms and of living areas, and not simply walk through without permission, or without connecting in a meaningful way to the people who live there. This concept is easier to grasp in household or small house models of care, where there is usually a door and a doorbell. In a traditional nursing home, elders' living areas are too often used as thoroughfares without any thought.

There are a variety of consultants with resources available for creating households out of traditional layouts, but these are beyond the scope of this book. Suffice it to say that large living areas can be segmented into "households" of 8 to 15 people, and many institutional trappings can be removed (such as nursing stations) with relatively minor renovation and expense.

Even in a small house, however, limits need to be set on exposure to strangers:

> St. John's Green House homes, by virtue of their unique placement in a residential community, have been a popular destination for visitors from around the world. In the first months after opening, there were many tours and visitations. But the strain of being an international "showcase" began to show on those who lived in the two houses.
>
> The staff held discussions with the elders in the houses, reaffirmed their Eden Alternative philosophy of nurturing close and continuous relationships, and found that the visitation process did not support this philosophy. Unfortunately, tours were too often a matter of people walking around and looking at the physical features, while paying little or no attention to those who lived there. Even when the elders and staff were acknowledged, it began to feel a bit like a "petting zoo."
>
> As a result, the houses now limit visits to about once a month, and the elders always give input on proposed visits and have the right to veto. There is no traditional tour; rather, all visits are set on the principle of engagement first (e.g., a luncheon or afternoon tea with the elders and staff); thus, the visitors get to see the home in the course of a primary social interaction. This has worked out much better, and has been a richer experience for the visitors as well.

St. John's Green House homes also proved instructive in helping sort out another recent question involving security:

> I was asked my opinion regarding Dutch doors, the kind that split in half, such that the lower half of the door can be closed while the upper half remains open. These are often proposed as a solution for living areas where there is a concern about people living with dementia who might walk into another person's bedroom uninvited.

There is no question that such an intrusion often causes anxiety for the person living in the room, but I still felt uncomfortable with the solution. While the person in the room could look out over the half door, it still seemed that it would function more as a way for others to look in, would not create the same degree of privacy as a closed solid door, and might even encourage others to try harder to get inside and look around.

I asked several people for their opinions. A couple of people noted the similarity of the doors to horse stalls, saying that they seemed undignified, while another said that they seemed preferable to stop signs and other artificial barriers being placed in front of rooms.

But in light of all we have discussed, there are reasons why people lose track of boundaries and feel like they are displaced; it seemed the problem went deeper. So I investigated the situation at St. John's Green House homes, where 10 people live in each house and most, but not all, have cognitive disabilities.

I learned that, while the elders have a strong sense of ownership of their home as a group (described earlier), there was not any significant intrusion into each other's bedrooms. Once again, the combination of a deinstitutionalized environment, the familiarity and connection, and the attention to individual rhythms, and to well-being in general, has created homes where the impetus to intrude has disappeared.

That observation has led me to conclude that such a transformation (both physical and operational) is the ideal solution because, rather than simply reacting to the intrusive actions, it eliminates the need for barriers in the first place. However, since this solution is not immediately available to all homes, this type of door might serve as a compromise, while the care partners continue to work on fulfilling the needs of those residing there.

Another physical/operational consideration when people enter others' rooms, particularly at night, is that most long-term care environments have compressed many of the activities of a resident's day into her sleeping space—watching television, reading, receiving visitors, and sometimes even eating meals. As a result, some people may look for another room at night because they are used to moving from these activities to a separate room for sleep. Helping create comfortable spaces outside the bedroom for these other activities may help in this regard, so that the bedroom becomes a true bedroom once again.

One other feature that the architects planned into St. John's Green House homes is a configuration that enables different degrees of engagement. The bedrooms are large and private, with a private toilet and shower. Outside of each cluster of rooms there is a small alcove, with seating available, before moving out into the common areas (living room and dining room). This enables people to choose how much they wish to engage with others, and gives those who are a bit hesitant a chance to "scope things out" before plunging into the mainstream.

While many more aspects could be addressed, I will close this chapter with a reminder that lighting and the acoustic environment are important components of security. These two aspects of the living environment were discussed in detail in *Dementia Beyond Drugs* (pp. 89–92) and should be reviewed because of their potential to have striking effects, positive or negative, on security as well as autonomy.

With regard to lighting, I will add here that nighttime illumination should be individualized to optimize each person's sense of security. Some people prefer some light in their sleeping environment, while others prefer complete darkness. For nighttime navigation to the bathroom, a small nightlight, floor illuminators, or a light triggered by a motion sensor may be useful. Also, examine the needs of staff when they enter rooms for nighttime care. How can they see enough to enter without throwing on a bright light that may frighten or annoy a sleeping person? There are many choices, from nightlights to small flashlights.

The audit of the acoustic environment suggested in *Dementia Beyond Drugs* (pp. 91–92) is good to revisit on a regular basis, as the sounds of institutional activity can creep into even the homiest environments. Recall that you are auditing not only for volume and unnatural sounds, but also the quality of other sounds (television, music), white noise from machinery, and the tone of voices when people speak.

These considerations are not limited to the nursing home environment. The sensitivity of people with cognitive disabilities (not only with dementia, but also with autism and other disorders) extends into all environments. Robert Simpson notes that he experienced similar problems in his community:

> You never realize until you see life through the eyes of an impaired person, howfastpeopletalktoeachother. Or how NOISY the world is, how stressful a walk around the block can be. The cacophony of voices, music, car horns. . . . When you are s-l-o-w to distinguish words and sounds, when it takes a conscious effort to sort them out, a city environment can be toxic. (Simpson & Simpson, 1999, p. 84)

I have come to see people living with dementia as akin to "canaries in the coal mine." In the early days of coal mining, canaries were carried into the mines because of their sensitivity to toxic gases. If a miner saw a dead canary in the cage, it was a warning to get out before the gases reached a level toxic to humans. People living with dementia often become extraordinarily sensitive to the acoustic milieu, and will become upset when many of us do not feel outwardly distressed.

But, just like the canary, such people are reacting to an environment that is ultimately harmful to all of us. Studies have shown that noisy, hectic environments can have effects on all people, even when we are unaware of it. Studies of sleeping participants subjected to environmental noise, such as traffic or jet aircraft, showed not only sleep and mood disturbances, but also increases in blood pressure, respirations, and adrenaline release, as well as changes in cardiac immune function, even when the subjects remained asleep (Haralabidas, A. S., Dimakopoulou, K., Vigna-Taglianti, F., et al., 2008; Schmidt, F. P., Basner, M., Kröger, G., et al., 2013; WHO, 2013) .

Some homes have used a decibel monitor with a light that illuminates above a certain volume level as a visual reminder when things get out of hand. Keep in mind, however, that it is not simply noise levels; a tense or defensive voice can have an equally bothersome effect. The lesson is that when people react to the sounds in their living environment, we should quickly move to change the sonic landscape they experience, for ourselves as well as for them.

Another important way to enhance security is to ensure that people have some degree of control over their surroundings. This leads us to the domain of Autonomy, and Chapter 6.

Autonomy

I live with the imminent dread that one mistake in my
daily life will mean another freedom will be taken from me.

—Robert Davis

The relative power of the aged vis-à-vis their social environment is gradually diminished until all that remains of
their power resources is the humble capacity to comply.

—James Dowd

If you want total security, go to prison. There you're fed,
clothed, given medical care and so on. The only thing
lacking . . . is freedom.

—Dwight D. Eisenhower

OF THE SEVEN DOMAINS of well-being described in this book, there is
none more treasured by people living with dementia, nor so hotly con-
tested, than autonomy. The ability to choose our life's path, to make
decisions large and small, even to make choices that we know may not
be in our best interest, is a fundamental human right. There is also no
other domain whose discussion demands a more critical inward look at
our own beliefs and values.

The United States of America was established after fighting a war
over autonomy. My hometown of Rochester, New York, is the burial
site of two local citizens who fought for autonomy—through the aboli-
tion of slavery (Frederick Douglass) and women's right to vote (Susan
B. Anthony). Many of our current political debates center on issues of

individual autonomy vis-à-vis the role of the government. And many other such movements have punctuated our history, and the histories of other nations around the world for millennia before our country existed.

The ability to vote, to have a voice in the affairs of our nation, is a right granted to all adult citizens of the United States, including those who lack formal education and those who live with a wide variety of physical and psychiatric disorders. One may also choose not to vote without sacrificing other rights of citizenship or the right to make a multitude of other day-to-day decisions.

When living with dementia, however, things get a bit more complicated. Questions of one's ability to make wise decisions are raised early and often, and extend far beyond the rights and responsibilities of citizenship to even the most mundane choices. As mentioned in Chapter 4, "poor judgment" is on display daily throughout society and well profiled in the media, particularly among celebrities and politicians; yet, if anyone were to suggest that such individuals surrender all decision-making capacity to others, there would be an outcry.

This is not to suggest that cognitive disorders do not erode certain capabilities. The question, however, is how to support people and where to draw the line. After all, a personality disorder that leads a public figure to live irresponsibly is never considered medical grounds for incapacity, while a diagnosis of dementia, more often than not, leads us to assume one's incapacity well before the fact.

Autonomy Defined

Fox et al. (2005) gave *autonomy* the defining characteristics of "liberty; self-governance; self-determination; immunity from the arbitrary exercise of authority; choice; and freedom." These terms encompass many aspects of autonomy: the ability to choose, the right not to be coerced or constrained, the right to monitor one's own actions (within the law), and the right to chart one's path through life.

As mentioned in Chapter 5, autonomy sits side by side with security in my rendering of the hierarchy of the Fox et al. (2005) domains in the well-being pyramid (Figure 3). There is continuous interplay between the two domains, sometimes in concert, sometimes in conflict. For example, a degree of emotional and physical security is needed to optimize autonomy. However, an overemphasis on physical and emotional safety can erode one's autonomy.

Therefore, the balance of these two domains becomes critical, if higher domains of meaning, growth, and joy are to be attained. This caveat also reflects former President Eisenhower's quote at the beginning of this chapter, and although he likely was referring to our collective security as a nation, the same can be said for the individual. (Eisenhower's quote is a restatement of an earlier quote—variously attributed to Founding Fathers Benjamin Franklin and Samuel Adams—that "people willing to trade their freedom for temporary security deserve neither and will lose both.")

So our well-being pyramid is not made entirely of stone. While the foundation layer of identity and connectedness may be relatively solid, the next level is fluid and shifting, and these shifts will influence the higher levels as well. In fact, I would argue that this is not a two-dimensional "pyramid," but a three-dimensional object, in which the third dimension represents the progress of the seven domains through the course of time. The reason is that time will affect one's cognitive and physical capabilities, and, therefore, the interplay of the seven domains (and the ways in which they are met) will necessarily shift as well.

How Dementia Challenges Autonomy

Intrinsic Challenges

The ability to choose or to make decisions is greatly affected when memory and procedural memory become challenged. Impaired memory also makes it difficult for people to call up the various options available for choices. A simple example is a person going to breakfast and being asked, "What would you like to drink?" and having difficulty generating a mental list of hot and cold beverages one might have with breakfast.

In addition to forgetfulness, people living with different forms of dementia often develop problems with executive function—the ability to plan, sequence, and problem-solve multistep tasks. My preference in this chapter is to place the many issues commonly referred to as "impaired judgment" (such as forgetting to wear a coat outside in cold weather) in this category. Doing so relates the problem to a set of planning and sequencing skills, rather than to a more subjective assessment of whether one is making an unwise decision (as many people without dementia may also do).

Another important barrier to autonomy results from challenges with language. Those who have trouble with word-finding or other aspects of verbal expression are often unable to exercise choice in a manner recognized by their care partners. (As we will discuss later, even those who are unable to speak are often expressing choice in ways that we fail to appreciate.) The inability to filter out competing sounds or other environmental stimuli is another impediment to making clear and focused decisions.

Being "unstuck in time" can lead to problems where decisions require a temporal framework for success and safety. Knowing how long to be exposed to heat, sun, or cold may be a factor in going outside safely; inattention to cooking times, medication times, or the appropriate time and distance to reach a destination may add to the risk of living alone, walking, or driving.

Finally, any physical challenges related to the type of dementia (or to age-related illnesses) may also be barriers to exercising choice and engaging in independent activity. Examples include peripheral vision loss related to Alzheimer's, rigidity due to Parkinsonism, or age-related hearing loss. Concomitant depression can also impair one's attention, focus, and decision making.

Once again, a discussion of risks to autonomy raises the specter of security as well. Each of the deficits just listed is more likely to become an issue when personal safety or the safety of others is at stake.

Extrinsic Challenges

The foregoing list of intrinsic challenges alone might seem to make the erosion of autonomy insurmountable for people with cognitive disabilities. Worse yet, there are a host of extrinsic challenges that further add to this burden. Just as we look at transforming personal, operational, and physical aspects of the living environment, we can see that autonomy is eroded significantly in each of these three aspects.

Personal Barriers

Intrapersonal and interpersonal barriers arise from our dominant view of dementia, beginning with the stigmatized view that the diagnosis renders a person incapable of making choices. This goes far beyond those living with forgetfulness, to the stigmas related to ageism in general. There is a tendency for younger adults to speak for their elders, even when there is no evidence of cognitive disability. Once again, our societal focus on doing (as opposed to being) leads us to assume that those who do less need others to guide them.

Bartlett and O'Connor (2010) remind us that "historically, there has been a tendency to accord family members higher credibility and responsibility around decision making, irrespective of whether this is warranted or not" (p. 55). They ask us to be mindful of the following questions in each discussion: "Whose voices are being heard? Whose voices are being silenced?" (p. 58).

> This aspect of ageism was made particularly clear to me one day while traveling on an airplane to give one of my talks. I overheard a man and woman making conversation in the row behind me. At one point, the gentleman mentioned that his parents were living in the community, but "they have arthritis and are slowing down, and my sister and I have decided we need to tell them it's time to move to assisted living." There was no mention of discussing his parents' concerns with them, looking for input, or recognizing their right to choose.
>
> The ageism was driven home even further when the woman asked the man how old his parents were. "Well," he replied, "my mother is only 62 but my father is nearly 66 years old." (I wonder what he'll consider their capabilities to be when they are 20 to 30 years older still?)

Since society already applies a fair degree of stigma to older adults in general, adding the cognitive changes of dementia makes it very easy for us to assume that such people are completely incapable of rational decision making. Once again, our tendency to use all-or-none thinking blinds us to the many nuances of autonomy, and as Kitwood described, we "position" people as being less capable than they are. The stigmas regarding one's identity and personhood outlined in Chapter 3 have once again come home to roost.

From an interpersonal standpoint, many types of disempowering interactions occur in all living environments. The 17 different aspects of "malignant social psychology" described by Kitwood (1997) have been extensively reviewed in many publications, including my first book. Examples of these interactions include deception (giving false or insufficient information in an attempt to redirect a person from an action or desire she is expressing), and outpacing (providing information too quickly or without giving adequate time for the person to process and respond, then assuming he cannot decide).

The ultimate danger of these interactions and the stigmas that cause them, once again, is the self-fulfilling prophecy. When we make such assumptions about people's capabilities, we disempower them, and their subsequent detachment and discouragement cause *excess disability*, thus fulfilling our lowered expectations. Examples of statements leading to such self-fulfilling prophecies are: "He cannot decide, so we will decide for him"; "She cannot do that herself, so we will do it for her"; "People with dementia cannot learn"; and "People with dementia can only receive care—they cannot give care to others."

Added to this is the complex interpersonal dynamic created by one's dependency on others, whether due to physical or cognitive disability. Lustbader (1991) chronicled this dynamic in her book, *Counting on Kindness: The Dilemmas of Dependency*. Part of this dynamic comes from the powerlessness of being unable to act on our own:

> The more dependent we are on the mercy of others, the more waiting we have to endure. Dependence and waiting eventually become synonymous. (p. 6)

There is also a sense of guilt associated with leaning on others for support:

> She has "all day," while her daughter has to "fit" the errand into an array of doings. Her daughter's presence is in demand, while her presence is vital to no one. Each minute of waiting that accumulates speaks this inferiority more loudly. (p. 7)

Dependency, therefore, creates an imbalance of *power* as well. Such a dynamic is often created without malice, but as a result of one's attempt to provide care according to the traditional view that positions the person with the "disease" as incapable, thus requiring a "caregiver" to "do for him."

Bartlett and O'Connor (2010) state it this way:

> Oppressive and discriminatory practices often have their foothold in the well-meaning, well-intentioned ideas of those least intending to do harm. (p. 53)

Further along in the text, they back this idea up with two other references:

As Fox (1995) notes, a personhood lens does not have the language for exploring the possibility that "caring" might sometimes have more to do with power and control than with values of trust and giving. . . . (p. 25)

The "cosy image of care as synonymous with love can serve to mask the control that operates in many relationships where one person is substantially dependent on another." (p. 47, quoting Swain, French, & Cameron, 2003)

Thus, compassion and care often contain elements of control due to a stigmatized view of the person as being helpless and therefore in need of someone to "take over and act in his best interest." This is a primary drawback of "person-centered care" as many people practice it; it becomes a paternalistic process that uses substituted judgment in many day-to-day choices. The fact that the decision may not match the wishes of the person with dementia is, to some extent, beside the point; the larger issue is the premise that there is no value to involving the person in the decision-making process in the first place.

And speaking of person-centered care, another fundamental barrier to autonomy in "long-term care" environments is exactly that—the equating of "living" with "care," such that the needs of the person are reduced to the physical, and life is medicalized. Medicalized living, in turn, increases the shadow of the "disease" looming over all aspects of the person's life, and the vicious cycle of self-fulfilling prophecies rolls on.

As such, Bartlett and O'Connor (2010), in a powerful text, argue that matters of choice must reach well beyond matters of everyday life and care to the level of social citizenship:

It is primarily about social, political and cultural dynamics, rather than individual clinical or social psychology. (p. 4)

Later, they provide a list of various complaints and concerns voiced by people living with dementia to reinforce the point:

Unfortunately, comments like these are rarely heard or interpreted in a political way. This is partly because clinical and psychosocial explanations of people's behaviours prevail, particularly in long-term care settings. . . . Yet narratives like these must be recognised for what they are, namely, an attempt to regain power and control. (p. 85)

In summary, a narrow biomedical view of dementia leads to disempowerment through stigma and positioning. But even more, the medicalization of the lives of such people further disempowers them by limiting the range of discussions and possibilities regarding their larger place in the social fabric. (I will return to the notion of social citizenship at the end of the book.)

Before we move on, there is a little-appreciated form of autonomy that was brought to my attention. While I was teaching a seminar in London, a participant asked me if we should also address the topic of *emotional autonomy*. That is, do people living with a diagnosis of dementia have the power to express their emotions freely, without judgment or disparagement?

A medicalized view of the person causes us to see an expression of anger or sorrow as the "emotional lability" of a damaged brain. Especially in nursing homes, we have an expectation that all must be tranquil, and we confuse the absence of emotional upset with well-being.

Indeed, people experience a range of emotions in the course of a normal life, and it is equally normal to express them. Yet, how often do tears or an angry outburst compel the staff to regard the situation as a "problem" to be remedied or brought to a quick resolution? Our intolerance for such emotions leads us to seek interventions, whether pharmaceutical or diversional, which will bring about such a resolution.

The medicalization of the condition blinds us to the realization that each of us experiences similar emotions, sometimes to an exaggerated degree:

> On a recent speaking trip, the passengers on my upcoming flight were informed that, due to a mechanical problem, our flight would experience a delay. One businessman in the gate area responded by walking over and accosting the gate agent with angry, sarcastic questions about whether they *ever* had a flight leave on time from this airport. The agent maintained her poise, and he eventually returned to his seat.
>
> A few minutes later, the agent announced that, due to the delay, they would be bringing another plane into service, but that it could take up to another hour to do so. The man cursed loudly and stormed out of the area to find other arrangements, kicking the trash can as he passed it. (In a delicious irony, the mechanical problem was resolved five minutes later, and we departed soon after, minus one angry passenger who did not bother to wait a bit longer.)

Having just delivered a series of talks on the topic of dementia, I could not help but be struck by the man's behavior, and considered what the likely response would have been if a person living in a nursing home had responded that way (e.g., after being told he could not go outside for a walk). In many instances, it would be added to the "behavior record" as further documentation of his poor judgment, emotional lability, and/or ongoing need for medication.

Every person needs to have the same autonomy of emotional expression that each of us has. On several occasions over the years, I have remarked to nursing home staff that "a person should be able to have a bad day once in a while without being given an antipsychotic." But the typical nursing home environment demands more perfection than most of us could muster in such surroundings. This, in turn, creates more stress for those who, already feeling a loss of autonomy, must conform to these expectations, even while living in institutionalized surroundings. Wong (2009) shared the observation of Albert Camus (in *Notebooks: 1942–1951*) that "Nobody realizes that some people expend enormous energy, just to be normal" (p. 160).

Operational Barriers

The primary ways in which people are disempowered through operational aspects of life and care are through the self-fulfilling prophecies described earlier. We disempower by doing for, deciding for, excluding from discussions, and creating regimented living schedules that place organizational priorities above personal choice.

These operational aspects are important to recognize, because care partners often take the blame for not being caring, compassionate, or having a work ethic, when in fact it is often the entrenched system of care that is the real culprit. In her brilliant paper, McLean (2007) describes the "cult of clock time and task" that drives most nursing home operations. Not only does the provision of care prioritize task completion over relationship, the system also compartmentalizes all aspects of life into artificial time periods that reflect the organization's need to complete those tasks, irrespective of how it affects those forced into such artificial rhythms. As the article's title states, McLean calls for "A return to the sanctity of 'lived time,'" and argues that much of the distress we see in nursing homes arises from the conflicts that such operational priorities cause (recall the Beatitudes Campus approach to "sundown syndrome" described in Chapter 3).

Further erosion of autonomy for people living in nursing homes (and assisted living as well) arises from the effect these time demands have on staff. Being forced into a task mentality does not give care partners the time or flexibility needed to empower people who may need a bit more time, or a bit more help, in order to make choices or do for themselves. As such, the person who is walking slowly to the dining room will be put in a wheelchair and whisked away to the meal; the person who takes more time to eat will have the fork taken away and be assisted with the meal; the person who must maneuver her arthritic fingers slowly to button a blouse will be summarily dressed instead; and the person who must work slowly to express himself verbally may be cut off or ignored, and decisions made on his behalf. And as the saying goes, if you don't use it, you lose it.

The institutional model of care can erode these domains of well-being for the *staff* as well, and autonomy is a prime example. In order for a care partner to empower her elders, she must, in turn, be empowered— to flex her time and tasks as her charges dictate, to make decisions in the moment that can help honor their requests, or to follow the diverse needs of a diverse population. Such empowerment is too often lacking, and there is a trickle-down effect for the people she serves.

While many homes aspire to provide "person-centered care," the truth is that departmental and organizational priorities nearly always trump the desires of the individual. One need only ask, "If an individual wants something that is inconvenient and requires some effort for the organization to accommodate, what is the likely outcome?" That is the true test of how person-centered we are, and few pass the exam.

Lastly, the embedded use of stigmatizing language is another operational challenge to empowerment. When one is labeled as "delusional," "agitated," "confused," or "acting out," it is far easier to discount her opinion and look to others to decide for her.

Physical Barriers

The traditional nursing home or assisted living community contains a wealth of structural impediments to autonomy. A major impediment, as seen with security, is that of the overall scale. A larger environment is more difficult to commit to memory for successful navigation, and the physical distance between various rooms can be daunting to people who have difficulty walking. Many people who had walked unaided in their smaller homes or apartments find themselves wheelchair bound, unable to manage the physical demands of living in a much larger space. They have become "functionally disabled."

Inadequate or inappropriate lighting and disturbing acoustics (related to volume, unexpected or artificial sounds, or competing sounds from a chaotic environment) challenge a person's ability to navigate, to think calmly and clearly, or to understand and be understood in conversations. These attributes are discussed in detail in Chapter 6 of *Dementia Beyond Drugs*, and, once again, the resonance with the domain of security is clear.

Other aspects of the physical environment serve to reinforce the power dynamic inherent in these environments. The nursing station forms a wall between the person and those who provide assistance, creating a physical barrier to contact and communication, as well as reinforcing the seat of power that lies with the organization. Some nursing stations are veritable fortresses.

In the course of her experiential nursing home thesis (described in Chapter 4), Dr. Emi Kiyota—living in the shoes of a nursing home resident—took photos of the environment from her wheelchair, to get an "elder's-eye view" of the living areas. One of her photos showed the front of the nursing station, the counter looming above her head. At the time she took the photo, she was conversing with a staff member behind the counter whose face was entirely shielded by the structure.

There is no need to repeat an exhaustive discussion of all the features of the traditional nursing home that we would never find in a real home. But one other aspect of the physical environment deserves mention: the array of features that serve to reinforce the "sick role" of those who live there, thus increasing dependence in very real ways.

In addition to the nursing station, medication carts preserve a hospital atmosphere, where the efficient dispensing of medications is the priority. This may help nurses bring pills to each person's room in the morning and evening, but at other times of the day it will often be positioned near the dining room or activity room, and medications administered as people enter or while they sit.

This has several deleterious effects. First, it medicalizes once-normal activities such as meals and social gatherings. Second, it brings the dose of medicine at a time that may or may not be ideal for the individual, but serves the institutional need to catch several people's doses at one time. The result of this homogenization of administration times might be having to swallow a large complement of pills before eating that could ruin anyone's appetite or taste for food; or taking a pill that leads to an untimely need to use the toilet; or a drop in blood pressure during an activity, often compounding the usual drop that accompanies digestion after a meal.

A third effect of the medication cart is the constant visual reminder of one's illness and need for pills. Many household- or small-house-style homes have eliminated their carts in favor of individual medication cabinets in each person's room. They often report a decrease in requests for medication for pain or anxiety, due to the elimination of the constant visible reminder of one's illness.

Another subtle, yet powerful trapping of the institution is the presence of uniforms and scrub clothes. This may seem like a minor point, but when those around you dress like people who tend to the sick, it is very difficult to see your potential for growth and positive engagement with life.

I heard the story of a Green House community where the staff expressed the desire to continue to wear uniforms and scrubs, and secured the agreement of the elders living in the home. But they stuck with their tradition of "dressing down" in street clothes on weekends. After several weeks, it became apparent that on the days when the staff wore their uniforms, the elders were more passive and dependent, while they were more likely to show initiative and independence on the weekends when the staff wore normal street clothes. A powerful message indeed. (From a personal communication, I learned that Suzanne Mumford of Hallmark Care Homes, U.K., is commissioning a study with Dr. Dawn Brooker of the University of Worcester to look at the evidence base for eliminating uniforms. I am very much looking forward to hearing the results of that study.)

> Another example of the subtle power of environment to reinforce the sick role is from St. John's Green House® homes. Before the homes opened, the new staff members were given cooking classes held in the homes. As a way to practice their skills, a group of elders and staff were invited over from the nursing home each day to enjoy a lunch prepared for them.
>
> Dave is a retired engineer who has a progressive dementia that also affects his ability to stand and his ability to speak fluently. At the nursing home, it had been a longstanding routine to have two staff members transfer him from one chair to another. Since he was to be one of the first residents of the new homes, he was invited to lunch one day with his family.

Dave was transported to the home via a wheelchair transport van and was then wheeled around his future home, so that he could see the house in which he would soon live. Then he was lifted to a chair at the communal dining room table and he, his family, staff members, and other visitors sat together for a relaxed and tasty lunch of soup and sandwiches, served on real china and enjoyed slowly, amid normal conversation.

At the end of a pleasant hour of convivium, it was time for Dave to return to his room at the nursing home. The staff brought the wheelchair over, but before they could move to help him, Dave stood up and transferred himself into the wheelchair. Rebecca, the administrator, came over and said, "Hey, Dave, what's going on? It takes two people to lift you to your chair at the nursing home!"

In his slow, halting speech, Dave replied, "I don't know. I guess over there, I'm supposed to be sick."

Many other physical features and trappings, such as alarms, bibs, and double rooms, can negatively affect autonomy as well. Clearly it would be a rare individual who could assert himself in institutional living, and anyone who did may well be viewed as a "problem."

Segregated Living and Autonomy

There are many potential barriers to autonomy in dementia-specific living environments. Many of these are identical to those already described, as stigmas, operational practices, and structural elements are often the same in both integrated and segregated communities. There are, however, some additional considerations when people living with dementia are separated.

The very philosophy that leads to segregated living is probably the biggest barrier to autonomy. People are most commonly moved to segregated living areas in order to be in a locked, alarmed area, or because they are expressing needs that are not able to be understood or met in their current setting. As a result, the decision to move the person is entirely dictated by the concerns of others (staff, other elders, or their families), and/or follows the preferences of the nursing home operators, regarding their own need to minimize their liability risk. In other words, such a move is driven by the desires of everyone *but* the person in question. It would be a rare day when a person living with dementia would advocate to be relocated to a locked unit. Therefore, by definition, such moves defy individual choice.

While the staff in many segregated living areas work hard to provide humane care and fight the stigmas seen with dementia, their efforts remain in fundamental conflict with a model that follows a stigmatized view of how people with dementia should live. It is much easier to fall prey to generalizations about the capabilities of people living with dementia when you work within a model that has already made generalizations about the type of living environment that they need.

Therefore, even exceptional care partners who work in segregated living areas must constantly resist the stigmas inherent in the philosophy of segregation. Conversely, while stigmas about dementia also exist in many integrated environments, it is easier to rise above such views when working within a model that houses people based on a fundamental philosophy of equality in living opportunities. Furthermore, working in an environment with people whose capabilities are more diverse would be expected to help one recognize and foster each person's individual potential.

Finally, as mentioned in Chapter 5, the presence of a lock and alarm in segregated areas creates a false sense of security for staff, who may not address the underlying causes of a person's attempts to leave. If staff do not pursue this line of critical thinking to identify and respond to the person's needs, his sense of autonomy is further eroded, along with his sense of security.

Community-Based Living and Autonomy

As discussed, the erosion of autonomy stems primarily from stigmatized, all-or-none views of the capabilities of the person living with cognitive disability. Stigmatized practices in nursing homes are reflective of larger societal attitudes that prevail in private homes as well.

The story of Ed Voris in Chapter 1 reminds us of the slippery slope of stigma and disempowerment that appears with the very mention of the word *Alzheimer's* or *dementia*. The quote by Robert Davis that opens this chapter is another example of the all-too-real threat to autonomy that awaits people who are diagnosed. In the same chapter, Davis (1989) elaborates further:

> Each freedom taken places me in a smaller playpen with a tighter ritual to maintain myself.
>
> For example, any housewife can forget a pan on the stove and burn dinner. She and her family just laugh about it and get a can

of something else out for supper. If a person with Alzheimer's gets caught burning something, it is a severe tragedy, another marker of the progress of her incompetency for self-sufficiency. In all likelihood, it will take away forever her opportunity to cook unless she has a very understanding, loving family who will allow her to cook but will be willing to keep an eye on the stove without her knowing it. For the healthy person, this will be just an honest mistake, but for the person with Alzheimer's, it may be the end to a whole line of productivity.

What fear this produces! (pp. 91–92)

Davis's comment not only captures the dread that this loss of choice and control brings, but also the irony of how a similar mistake made a few weeks before the diagnosis (or in a person without a diagnosis) would be seen in a completely different light. His opening line above also captures the infantilization felt by those who have had choice taken away from them. (Shortly before typing these words, I destroyed a teakettle by putting water on to boil, becoming immersed in my work, and forgetting about it until after the water had all boiled away. I do not, to my knowledge, have Alzheimer's, but it is a sobering reminder of how tenuous our rights are when the diagnosis appears.)

"A Meeting of the Minds" is a monthly webinar series hosted by Laura Bowly of Mindset Memory Centre in Vancouver, Canada, that convenes conversations among people living with dementia and those who support them. A group of participants living with dementia recorded one of their online support group conversations and then used the contents to create a dramatic reading, entitled "To Whom I May Concern." During the reading, one participant, Mike, shared his technique of engaging new acquaintances in conversation:

I have what I call my Ten-Minute Rule. . . . Whenever I meet someone, I always have a regular conversation. For the first ten minutes, I want them to know me, see that I'm normal, and then I might tell them I have Alzheimer's disease. If you did that right away, they'd immediately discount you. (Bowly, 2013)

Many people agonize over the resistance a family member shows when pressed to relinquish an activity such as driving. Exploring the domain of autonomy teaches us that often the resistance may not be specifically about the car. The person may well realize that he is having more trouble driving, but he is also all too aware of the slippery slope on which he stands. And he knows that giving up one bit of control may put him on a fast track to losing it all.

The power dynamics surrounding dependency play out in one's relationships with family and friends in the community as well. Often even the most tenuous connection to control is denied, so complete is the assumption of choice by one's family members. Lustbader (1991) wrote of visiting a man whose stroke had rendered him unable to speak or write. Because of his inability to say what he needed, he had been denied the opportunity to walk to the local store or otherwise engage his neighborhood independently. When Lustbader tried to interview him directly with yes-or-no questions, his wife repeatedly interrupted and answered the questions for him. Lustbader noticed that the man kept slapping his back pocket and pointing at his wife:

> Then I understood. "Your wallet. Where is your wallet?" I asked. He pointed more vigorously at his wife. "Oh," she said, "I'm storing it in his desk. He doesn't need it any more." (p. 19)

While the fact of his disability was undeniable, his wife failed to recognize the symbolic importance of keeping his wallet with him. The wallet was a metaphor for his ability to make choices and likely an extension of his masculinity as well. In fact, with proper guidance, he might well have been able to silently choose and purchase items at the neighborhood store, thus preserving a sense of meaning and importance.

Lastly, as implied earlier in the chapter, it is difficult to stand up and speak out without being branded a troublemaker, or having your advocacy seen as an abnormal emotional outburst. In the video "To Whom I May Concern," Steve laments that his advocacy to start a support group for people living with early-stage Alzheimer's branded him a "hard-ass" among those at his local support organization. Jeanne agrees that their advocacy puts them in a bind:

> We're not supposed to get angry; we're supposed to be on the receiving end of the care. Getting angry just doesn't fit the image of a "sick person." . . . We're supposed to be quiet and grateful. We're a burden. We've upset people's lives; we are the destroyers of the Golden Years of our spouses. Our kids are all set to switch places and become the parent. (Bowly, 2013)

Another participant, Joyce adds:

> I'm afraid I'll lose support if I share my frustration. I feel like I have to hide those feelings. (Bowly, 2013)

This hearkens back to the topic of emotional autonomy described earlier. Lustbader (1991) quotes a disabled man who was unable to vent his frustrations without repercussions:

> I soon learned that it was considered bad form for me to behave like a normal person in certain circumstances. (p. 112)

There is no question that our stigmatized view of dementia makes it hard for a person to speak out and truly be heard. After a particularly challenging appearance on a radio call-in show, Diana Friel McGowin (1993) made this observation:

> I have learned another lesson from this incident (and they say [Alzheimer's disease] patients cannot learn!). I have learned that when you stand up to be counted, you make a dandy target. (p. 136)

Enhancing Autonomy

Just as we discussed how autonomy is eroded through personal, operational, and physical barriers, we can use a similar framework to help find ways to safely restore choice and control.

Personal Transformation

In order to enhance autonomy, the most important first step is to make a shift in our own perception. This begins by abandoning all-or-none thinking about the issue, and realizing that autonomy, like security, occurs on many levels. We then must embrace the notion that life with dementia is not purely a deterioration of abilities. While some skills may be lost, others may actually become more acute, and still others may fluctuate—depending upon the day, the environment, or the facilitative skills of the care partner.

This shift also requires that we expand our thinking about what constitutes empowerment. We tend to think in terms of big decisions, and when these become too difficult, we assume that there is a lack of "competence." But competence is a legal concept that falls into the all-or-none arena of court hearings. A better way to look at autonomy is through the lens of *capacity*: the ability to make any given single decision.

Capacity can vary, depending upon the type of decision, the way in which choice is offered, and even the time of day. For many decisions, and for most people living with cognitive disability, capacity is not purely a yes-or-no determination. In fact, most people living with dementia can make decisions on *some* level, when given the chance, so it is important to add nuance to the concept of autonomy. Another concept that parallels our discussion of security is that small steps make a big difference in enhancing autonomy as well. And each of our three forms of transformation will help to bring this about.

The first rule for engagement is to approach the person with an open mind. Many ethical guidelines regarding people with developmental disabilities revolve around the presumption of capacity; that is, the person is assumed to be capable until he demonstrates that he is not. How different that is from the way in which we often view people living with dementia!

While it can be obvious that people with more severe disability cannot do certain things, it is always best to err on the side of presuming that they can do more than we may think. If they stumble repeatedly, then we will have an idea of their limits, but we can also feel confident that we probably did not sell them short.

The "care partner" concept (Power, 2010, p. 83) is another important mindset with which to approach the relationship. Rather than the one-way relationship of caregiving, the care partner image opens our mind to engaging in partnership with the person in the various decisions of everyday life, even if only informing him or checking for understanding before proceeding.

Taylor (2011) tells us that he needs "to be *enabled* and *re-abled.*" By *enabled* he means that there are some tasks and choices that are more difficult for him now; we should not take them over, but instead give the cues and assistance he needs to complete them in partnership with us. By *re-abled* he means that there are some tasks and decisions that he can still do, but that have been co-opted by his care partners to the point where he has lost the knowledge that he can still do them. He needs reminders of these preserved abilities that have been stifled by the care environment, so that they can be reawakened.

Communication as Empowerment

From an interpersonal standpoint, there is no interaction too small to have an impact on the domain of autonomy. Let us start with communication. At its most basic level, good communication is empowerment. If a person struggles in such areas as memory, focus, or verbal expression, then she will have trouble communicating her needs and desires. Therefore, it follows that a care partner with good "face-to-face" skills will empower her, whereas one without these skills will dis-empower her, because it will be harder for her to make choices if she cannot communicate them to others.

Many details regarding communication and facilitation can be found in *Dementia Beyond Drugs*, with some added information in Chapter 4 of this book. There is no need to repeat the information here, but that should not understate its importance. Autonomy starts and often ends with these face-to-face encounters. Again, I will stress the importance of being centered and present in the moment, focusing your attention on the person. Many people living with dementia can sense your lack of attention, and that can shut down their attempts to communicate with you. Furthermore, your presence helps you to better understand their verbal and nonverbal expressions, and to catch important clues.

Careful attention to the way in which we pose questions can also empower people who have difficulty expressing themselves. In addition to the communication tips shared previously, a narrative approach can be a powerful way to help people express more complex feelings related to their experiences:

> St. John's Green House homes in Penfield, New York, had an annual state survey, followed closely by a federal survey. Although they were found to be free of deficiencies, the follow-up survey was very burdensome and intimidating to staff and elders alike. The level of anxiety of several people living with dementia was heightened by over a week of intense scrutiny by a surveyor who seemed unaware of the effect her tone of questioning and body language were having on them.
>
> When the survey was over, administrator Rebecca Priest felt that it would be a good idea to "debrief" the experience with the people living in the home; but she also knew that some of the people had trouble expressing themselves verbally, especially in response to direct questioning. She reflected on an interaction she had regularly with her two young daughters, who would often process difficult emotions through a story. So at times they would say to her, "Mom, tell me a story about . . . ," as a way of approaching these experiences.
>
> Based on this insight, Priest held a conversation with the elders, in which she began by asking one of them, "Bob, tell me a story about a time when you faced a challenging situation." What followed from the group was an outflow of personal experience, wisdom, and, ultimately, healing.

Working through Tasks and Choices

After good communication skills, the next level of empowerment involves helping people work through tasks and express choices in everyday life. The key is to shift our perspective from the notion of doing *for* to doing *with*.

For personal care, it would be appropriate to revisit the acronym *SEE* described in my first book. The "S" stands for *slow down*. When care partners speak or move too quickly, a person who needs time to process and participate can become disempowered, and her subsequent feeling of loss of control often underlies angry outbursts. The first "E" stands for *engage*. Your care will be felt in a much more authentic and affectionate way if you are relating to the whole person during the task, rather than silently doing bodywork. As mentioned in Chapter 4, this is an ideal time to share stories and create strong relationships without adding any time to one's busy schedule.

Even when the person seems to be nonverbal, the act of speaking to her, sharing stories, and explaining each step of the process can enhance her feelings of trust and security and give her a better sense of being in control. Our words often penetrate more deeply than we imagine:

> A woman who attended one of my workshops told the story of working as a volunteer in a nursing home and visiting a woman with severe cognitive disability. The woman had been nonverbal since her arrival, and it was assumed that she was also unable to comprehend others. The volunteer would nevertheless talk to her during her visits and tell her about herself and her family, and sometimes she would hold her or sing to her.
>
> After several months of periodic visits, the volunteer's husband received an out-of-town job transfer, and so she had to leave the nursing home and her friend. On her last visit, she lay next to the woman, held her, and explained that she was moving away and would not be visiting anymore. As she spoke, she saw a tear roll down the woman's cheek.
>
> Surprised, she asked the woman if she understood what she was saying. The woman nodded and spoke a hoarse "yes." She asked her if she had been able to speak all along, and the woman answered in the affirmative. The volunteer asked her why she had not talked to others over all these months, and the woman replied, "No one ever took the time to ask me."

The second "E" stands for *empower*. Ask yourself how the person can direct or give input to the process, even if she cannot do it all by herself. During a bath or shower, for instance, one could have the person direct the order of proceedings and indicate what she would like to do for herself and what may require some assistance. Repeated checks for comfort (e.g., "How is the water temperature? Does it need to be warmer? Cooler?") help the person know that she still has the ability to give input that you will follow.

Another aspect of "empower" is not only explaining each step that you are about to take, but also pausing to ensure there is understanding *and* acceptance before proceeding. Many care partners have been the target of angry words or gestures during personal care. They may wonder why this happened: "I told her I was going to rinse her hair before I did it." But it is not enough to say the words; they must be comprehended, and the person should give a sign that she is ready and accepting, or it may still come to her as an unwanted surprise.

Note that in the last paragraph, I recommend gaining consent for *each* step in the care process. Greenwood (personal communication, September 2, 2013) uses the term *continual consent*, reminding us that consent can be affected by short-term memory and attention distractors, so giving a single consent for a shower may not imply that the consent will be automatic for each stage of the process.

Choice can also be enabled through our wording, or by framing the options in a way that the person can process successfully. Earlier in the chapter, I gave the example of a person who could not mentally produce a list of drink choices at breakfast when asked in an open-ended way. If this happens, breaking the list into fewer choices can better enable him to choose a preference. One could start with the hot beverages ("Would you like coffee or tea?") then add cold drinks ("Orange, apple, or tomato juice?"), and so on.

When verbal expression is more challenged, Jane Verity (2010) of Dementia Care Australia suggests a combination of verbal and visual cues, along with simplified sentences that drop unimportant words and give a slight emphasis to the key words in the phrase. For example, one could hold a cup of coffee in one hand and tea in the other, presenting them one at a time, with the words, "Mary, *today*, will it be *coffee* or *tea?*"

The combination of verbal and visual cues often helps a person with language difficulties, and even if she is unable to speak, Mary may be able to point, nod, or smile, indicating her preference. The use of a person's name is often a good way to refocus her attention, which may be distracted; a light touch on the arm along with the stated name can help as well.

This graduated approach to tasks can be used in any situation, until the ideal level of enabling is identified. Another example might be brushing someone's teeth. For many people, a reminder to brush their teeth may be sufficient. Others may need help putting the toothpaste on the brush, or verbal and/or visual cues.

In cases where the person still seems unable to start brushing, using a "hand-in-hand" technique to start the brushing action is often sufficient to reawaken the memory of the activity. Holding the person's hand in yours also gives tactile feedback to ensure that the pace and pressure of the brushing are not excessive. At all of these levels, the person is involved to some extent, rather than a care partner simply doing the task for her.

As mentioned in *Dementia Beyond Drugs*, be aware of three areas where many people living with dementia often get "stuck": initiating an activity, sequencing the steps properly, or problem solving if the task does not turn out as planned. Giving appropriate cues can help the person through each of these barriers.

The same principles can be applied to any activities or tasks throughout the day. For a person who feels a loss of autonomy, there are no acts too small to be of benefit with this type of approach. The sum of all of these small empowering actions will be a far greater sense of control.

In long-term living environments, two areas in which people often assert themselves involve taking medications or going down the hall for a shower or bath. While care partners should review these processes in detail to find out how they might be done better, there may be a larger issue at stake. What the person may actually be saying is that there is *no* choice available to him throughout the day. So he exerts control in the places where it is easiest to do so; namely, he can easily decide to clamp his mouth shut and not swallow a pill, or to resist going down the hall to the shower room. When we realize that these expressions may indicate a larger issue with autonomy in general, we can begin to empower the person throughout the little interactions and choices of the day. When we do so, the big "No" around showers or pills often disappears, because the deeper need has been met.

Another key to enabling autonomy is finding the proper choice of words to communicate a task. Saying, "Please use the toilet now" may not give enough direction, whereas, "Pull your pants down; now sit down there" may provide the cueing that works better. Remember the "word palette" from Chapter 4, and keep in mind that different people may respond to different language choices.

In cases where people seem to resist your suggestions, a more collaborative approach is usually far more successful. Camp (2012) provides examples of this technique:

> If you are a woman caring for a woman with dementia, one approach to bringing her to the bathroom is to say, "Why don't we go and powder our noses?" . . . Another option is to say something like, "I have a great shade of lipstick that would look wonderful on you. Let's go and try it on together." The key is to make this an invitation to a social exchange rather than a command situation or a way of controlling the older adult. (p. 112)

In her memoir, Shanks (1999) relates the story of a telling comment made by her husband after she removed his clothes for a bath in a rather brusque manner, and the insight she gained for a more affectionate approach: "One time in the early years, after I had struggled to get all his clothes off, he stood nude, sadly shaking his head: 'Now, I don't have anything,' he said" (p. 54).

Her solution was to start the process in the living room, while he sat on his favorite couch, by giving him a foot massage, removing his shoes and socks in the process. As the massage continued, he relaxed and began to allow her to gradually remove more clothing and move him to the bath. On cold nights, she often began with a footbath in warm water, which was also very relaxing for him.

Once again, the key to all of the above approaches is to shift from *doing for* to *doing with*. **S**low down, **E**ngage, **E**mpower. (Readers of my first book may note that I have changed the order of the two "E's." Dr. Nader Shabahangi made the astute observation to me that engagement needs to come first if we are to understand how to truly empower the person.)

Choice without Words

What about people who have greater impairments or may be unable to express themselves verbally? It is crucial to understand that they still express choice through their actions. Instead of framing such actions as "behavior problems," look at the person as exercising choice, and new insights may appear. Although this is not always easy to do, if a care partner can step back from a resistant person and think, "What is he teaching me right now about my approach?" she can often discover how better to interact and eliminate the distress. As a person living with Alzheimer's, Voris (Voris, Shabahangi, & Fox, 2009) echoes this approach:

> Just think for a moment: how does your attitude change if you know you are approaching someone you think is your teacher versus if you are approaching someone you think is diseased, cognitively impaired? . . . A central question becomes: How would you like to be approached if you were forgetful? What would you like the eyes to see that look at you? (p. 119)

Many care partners are so task-oriented that they tend to push through resistance, just to "get it over with." This usually has a deleterious effect and leaves an indelible emotional memory that will make future care more difficult as well.

> At a symposium that we shared, psychologist Kort Nygard (2012) told the story of a woman who was regularly striking out at the nursing home staff during personal care. Unable to solve the problem, they hired a consultant to observe her for a day and make suggestions. After a day's observation, the team met with the consultant in a conference room, eager to hear all that she might have to offer.
>
> The consultant addressed the team as follows: "Here is what I have learned: when she raises her hand, palm up like this" (she demonstrated), "it means 'stop.'" End of consultation. The staff had been so fixated on getting the job done that they had missed her obvious attempts to tell them that the pace and approach were distressing her, so when they pressed on, she reacted physically.

It is also important to remember that lower levels of capability do not necessarily preclude all decisions about care. While the biomedical approach tends to evaluate cognition as a series of discrete tasks, people may possess integrated knowledge, logic, or wisdom that belies their Mini-Mental State Examination score. For example, a person may not remember the time or place, but she may be perfectly capable of giving a consistent, nuanced opinion about her desire to forgo life-saving measures, should the need arise.

Once again, the rule should be to presume capacity and discuss the decision with the person, to see if she can offer an opinion that is consistent and shows a process of reasoning behind it. Keep in mind that it does not have to reflect what we (or her family) think is best in order to be valid. Also, remember that one's capacity can fluctuate. A person may be more confused early or late in the day, or when distressed by a noisy environment, yet still be able to focus and make durable decisions at other times.

Finally, a person can change her mind. We all do, from time to time. What is more important is evidence of the thought process behind the change. Sometimes, even a person who appears to have no capacity to give input can express himself in a manner that helps care partners to make important decisions on his behalf:

> In *Inside Alzheimer's* (2007), Nancy Pearce tells the story of "Robert," a very proud and independent man who, in a late stage of Alzheimer's, was not taking in enough nutrition to sustain himself. Most of the food that was offered was pocketed in his cheeks, or dribbled down his chin. A family meeting was called, and even though he seemed unable to speak or comprehend, his daughter, Liz, knowing his history of always wanting to be in charge, suggested that they meet in Robert's presence, in case there was any way he could signal his understanding.
>
> The physician carefully explained Robert's clinical situation, but Robert stared blankly, without showing signs of comprehension. His daughter asked him some questions directly, such as whether he would want to use intravenous antibiotics in case of infection, but he continued to show no response.
>
> The doctor then began to tell Robert's daughter about the option of a gastrostomy tube to feed Robert, and described the procedure. "Suddenly, Robert began rocking back and forth in his chair, his brow furrowed, his eyes open and his breathing twice the rate of what it had been. We had to ask ourselves, why now?" (p. 241)
>
> The connection seemed to be related to the feeding tube discussion, so the group checked and rechecked throughout the afternoon, alternatively discussing various options in Robert's presence. "The only times Robert consistently showed agitated reactions were those when we mentioned placement of a G-tube. By day's end, we were convinced that he was quite clearly making his wishes known, even though our rational minds did not ever dream this would have been possible considering his level of confusion. When Liz told him that we would not talk any more about it and that the G-tube would not be inserted, Robert breathed that familiar long, deep and comforting sigh. We honored what we all knew was his wish." (pp. 241–242)

This is a remarkable story, not just because Robert was able to comprehend the meaning of the G-tube insertion, but also because his care partners had the awareness and sensitivity to respond to his signals, verify them beyond reasonable doubt, and act on them with regard to critical end-of-life decisions. People who might have considered him "incompetent" to make such a decision could have easily discounted his reactions. Worse yet, how many "Roberts" are out there who are never given the chance to attend such discussions, nor have the opportunity to express themselves, because we assume they are unaware?

Enhancing Emotional Autonomy

Finally, let us return to the concept of emotional autonomy. How can we help people to express the full range of human emotions in a way that is supportive and not stigmatizing? The first step is to understand that they occur, and that no living environment can eliminate feelings of sadness and anger that occur due to life's challenges and experiences.

This is another reason why we should always approach the person in distress by first naming and validating the distress we see. If we begin simply by saying "Calm down," or "Don't cry," or by challenging the reality of the feeling they are expressing, then we have denied them the right to have a full range of feelings. Validation says, in effect, "It is your right to feel the way you do, without judgment or blame."

Such validation should be followed by attentive listening, helping the person explore his feelings and providing a needed release. Such expressions can also give valuable clues as to what caused his distress, so that challenges to well-being can be identified and can guide his wellness plan. While some people's losses may seem insurmountable, we should still feed the well-being domains as best we can. So even though, for example, we cannot bring back a spouse who is deceased, we can provide loving companionship, connectedness, and security, and help the person find meaning and joy in celebrating the life they shared.

Operational Transformation

A system that focuses primarily on time and tasks is probably the biggest impediment to autonomy. This is because empowerment requires that we adjust our pace and routine to the ability of the person with cognitive disabilities. Even though the improvement in well-being may ultimately ease our burden of care in the long run, such an approach necessitates the devotion of extra time and flexibility at the outset. Organizations that cannot adjust their operations to better suit individual needs and rhythms will never succeed in enhancing this domain.

Bartlett and O'Connor (2010) concur:

> Good intentions alone are not adequate; promoting and valuing participation also means ensuring adequate resources are in place to allow a process to unfold that may take longer and be more complicated. (p. 72)

While the concept may seem onerous for an organization whose staff already feels overburdened, the long-term payoff is healthier people who are much less distressed, which in turn leads to greater family satisfaction, less staff burnout, and likely improvements in other health parameters as well. The key, just as with elimination of alarms, is to take small steps. Begin by adjusting to meet small needs in a small number of people and thereby gradually shift the operational dynamic. There will be a flywheel effect—the process will gain momentum as each operational shift provides a foundation on which the next may be more successful.

An example might be to find out people's preferred times for waking up in the morning and individual preferences for morning routines. Begin with just a few people, perhaps even one, and find a way to meet that person's preferred schedule and routine. When this is successful, choose one or more others. Organizations who follow this practice find a cumulative learning curve that smooths the process as it goes along, as well as a marked improvement in the demeanor of those in their care, which adds to the ability of care partners to make further shifts and receive positive results for their efforts.

Another key to this process is to work as seamlessly as possible across days and hours. This requires that we try to eliminate the "shift" mentality and consider all those who serve each individual as a single collaborative team, working together to meet her needs across the span of each day and night. Managers have a key role in fostering this team spirit and discouraging any dialogue that tries to separate or point fingers at different groups of people.

All of the approaches mentioned, from body language to communication skills to the various techniques to enable choice, must be taught and followed consistently across the team as well. This is a large enterprise that takes time and attention, but building this solid skill base will create better approaches that begin to happen automatically, and new arrivals will benefit from the day they move in. One day, someone may remark, "We don't see people trying to exit (or striking out, or calling out constantly) like we used to."

Negotiated Risk

In all living environments, the concept of negotiated risk (introduced in Chapter 5) is central to any form of empowerment, from employees and volunteers to people living with cognitive disabilities. But it is the latter group that raises most of the liability concerns, the focus on downside risk, and the tendency toward surplus safety.

As with our discussion of security, the best way to start is by creating autonomy in the multitude of small day-to-day actions and interactions, as outlined throughout this section. Starting small has the advantage of beginning with situations of low downside risk, thus helping the person to find success while increasing our comfort with the process of negotiating risk, and helping us to move away from all-or-none thinking.

Also, as already mentioned, many conflicts over large decisions come from the person's knowledge that giving up one decision may lead to a slippery slope of disempowerment. These smaller steps restore some of the autonomy that had been lost, and reassure the individual that his care partners will look at each new issue with fresh eyes and not paint him with the broad brush of "incompetence."

Negotiating risk involves several steps:

1. *Discussion.* This needs to be held directly with the person, to the extent that he is able to participate. All of the facilitation skills outlined previously should be employed to be sure that issues are understood as completely as possible, thus improving his opportunity to make the best choice.

2. *Exploration of values.* There are few absolutes with risk. Each decision to take a course of action is a combination of potential risk, potential benefit, and an understanding of how the person balances those two, based on his values and goals for the remainder of his life.

3. *Conditions of empowerment.* In culture change classes, we teach that successful empowerment requires five conditions: information, guidelines, skill development, additional resources, and a supportive environment. These should be reviewed to determine how a person could be best prepared to succeed. We also need to

consider specific challenges related to the individual and his illness, and explore ways to minimize the effect of these challenges.

4. *Continuum of empowerment.* There are many levels at which a person might exercise choice, as determined by considerations 1 through 3.

5. *Collaborative decision.* A final determination should be reached in as collaborative a fashion as possible.

6. *Monitoring results.* An ongoing monitor of how things are going will give feedback as to how well the plan was crafted, and may suggest adjustments to the plan as well. Also, people's capabilities can change over time, and so the plan may need to be revisited and amended.

7. *Keeping stakeholders abreast of the process.* Even when it is determined that the person has the right to make a choice, it is worth keeping family members, professional care staff, nursing home regulators, and others in the loop throughout discussions and documentation; not so that they can veto the decision, but so they can understand the process and share their own perspective.

Personal narratives can be very helpful in guiding discussions around negotiated risk. Just as a financial planner seeks to understand individual tolerance for risk, this information helps us understand the personal values of the individual seeking greater autonomy. Greenwood (personal communication, October 26, 2013) shared two stories of people she has known, showing the importance of this narrative:

> Joan lived a quiet mostly uneventful life (by choice) and lived in the same house her entire life. She never married, and looked after her sick mother until she died. She worked as a milliner in the same factory for 42 years, never drove a car, and attended the same church her entire life. She very rarely ventured out past her usual shopping areas, and was distraught when her favourite shop changed hands back in 1965.

> Harry worked as a builder. He actually scaled some of the highest buildings in Melbourne as they were being constructed. He likes to drink red wine—lots of it—and moved around Australia constantly looking for new adventures. Freedom was very important to him.

These examples beautifully illustrate the value of narrative in helping us understand how individuals' histories may influence how they balance autonomy with risk. Remember that the decision does not need to be what you or I would decide, nor does it need to be risk-free. But it must come from a discussion guided by the individual's goals and values, and the person's thinking process should have an internal consistency with regard to reflecting the values he has expressed.

For example, a person may request resuscitation in the case of cardiac arrest, even though we feel the likelihood of survival is very small, as long as he is consistent regarding his wishes, and supportive statements about his values indicate that he is willing to face low odds of survival in order to extend his life. On the other hand, a person who states that she does not wish to be kept alive with heroic measures, but then requests each and every life-saving option offered, shows an internal inconsistency that may lead one to question her capacity to continue to guide these directives.

Keep in mind that, even if the second person is incapable of choosing such directives, she may still be able to supply meaningful input about her values that could guide her agent(s) to act in concert with those values. And there are likely to be a multitude of other day-to-day decisions that she is still perfectly capable of making.

It is also important to understand that setting parameters or guidelines is not inconsistent with empowerment; all choice has limits. That is how we create the best balance of upside and downside risk. Returning to the somewhat controversial area of driving that was mentioned in Chapter 5, here is how Robert Davis (1989) created his own guidelines in order to avoid giving up driving completely:

> So far my physical response time has not been greatly affected. My great problem has been that of getting lost. Therefore, I limit my driving to a small radius around my home unless someone is with me to give directions. I also limit myself to driving only when I am well rested and feeling alert. (p. 92)

For those whose driving raises some concerns, but without gross evidence of unsafe practice, exploring parameters such as these can help improve the margin of safety without a complete abdication of all rights. (Assessing concerns regarding one's focus and attention may be a bit more difficult for family members. There are many older driver assessment programs that are skilled in making such evaluations.)

Once, during a "Meeting of the Minds" discussion, Dr. Richard Taylor was asked, as a person living with Alzheimer's, how he thought family members should handle concerns about a father who was not paying his bills correctly, but was resistant to turning over the control of his finances to a son or daughter. Taylor responded that a collaborative approach was likely to work better than simply taking the checkbook away completely.

He suggested a scenario in which the family member could express his desire to learn his father's bill-paying routine, "in case the time should come when I might need to do it for you." Taylor then outlined how the son could ask to sit with his father during the bill-paying sessions, to observe his system and learn what he needed to know in the future. In this manner, the father would continue to lead the process of bill paying, but the son could look over his shoulder and provide gentle guidance or reminders if he saw errors or omissions. Over time, his guidance might build his father's trust in his motives, and possibly also show his father that indeed he does need assistance.

In fact, it is often the abrupt removal of autonomy, or the threat thereof, that increases the potential for a crisis reaction:

> One evening, shortly before a community talk I was giving in Ohio, a local newswoman interviewed me. They had set up a live feed so that she could interview me at the venue where I was speaking. With the camera rolling, I began to answer a series of the "usual questions" that I am commonly asked. Then she threw a bit of a curveball.
>
> The reporter mentioned that a man with Alzheimer's had left his home in the community the day before and could not be found. She wondered what insights I might have about such a situation.
>
> As I paused to answer, several thoughts flashed through my mind: that I did not know the details of the situation, that I should be careful not to point blame at any individual, that people should not take such an episode as license to turn people's homes into prisons. But looking through the lens of the well-being domains, to me this was all about autonomy. So carefully choosing my words, I ventured the following answer:
>
> "Sometimes when people feel that they are losing all control over their lives, they can have a crisis reaction, where they simply try to escape and exert some independent control over their surroundings. That is why it is always good to partner in care with people living with dementia, and not simply decide everything for them."

> The reporter thanked me for my time, and I went on to my talk, wondering how many different ways my off-the-cuff comment might come back to haunt me. I did not stay up for the late news, and the next morning I gave two more talks for the local Alzheimer's Association chapter.
>
> During the lunch break, the executive director of the chapter mentioned to me that the man who had left his home had been found, and that he was safe. I told him that it was a great relief, and asked if there was any more information regarding what had happened. He replied, "Yes, apparently he had found out that his family was holding a court hearing the next day to assume guardianship."

Physical Transformation

There are many adjustments to the physical environment that can help enhance autonomy. The first is to keep the scale as small as possible. It is easier to memorize the layout of smaller living areas, and they are easier to navigate independently if one's strength and endurance are limited. In addition, we have described how a smaller environment can enhance security. As a general rule, one is more willing and able to be autonomous if one feels secure in his environment. It can also be helpful to include choice in the design, giving people options to engage in different areas, engage the same area differently, or reach the same area in different ways.

Even in one's own home, some limiting of the lived environment may improve both autonomy and security. Shanks (1999) describes several home modifications that helped her husband to feel, and be, more safe and assured. She kept certain doors closed, thus limiting his mental map of the house and empowering successful navigation. In addition to nailing the door to the bedroom closet shut (see Chapter 5), Shanks also positioned her husband's bed so that, when he got up, there was a direct path into the bathroom, which helped prevent him from getting misdirected and urinating in the wrong place.

Other wayfinding cues can be helpful, but usually need to be individualized. I have found that a generic system of guideposts in a nursing home may only work for some of those who live there, again because a one-size-fits-all approach may fall short. In addition to lettering and numbers, recognizable symbols also help to broaden the range of comprehension. Also, it is worth repeating that such cues are usually devised to compensate for a living space that is too large or too institutional to provide easy navigation. No such signage exists in St. John's Penfield Green House homes. People know where they are.

When signage is needed, it is important that the font size, lettering style and color, and placement on the walls are proper for people to visualize and comprehend. My colleague, Dr. Emi Kiyota, and I have visited a number of homes and hospitals where this is not the case. On a recent visit to the World Bank, we noted that the meeting room signs had a very stylish, modern, shiny gray-on-gray lettering and background that was almost impossible to read, even for us. Hopefully there are few people with 80-year-old eyes trying to navigate those hallways alone.

Camp (2012) reminds us that even people with dementia who have trouble with speech are often able to read. It is something we often do automatically, without even realizing that the words have registered. Written instructions can be helpful aids to comprehension, even for people with more advanced disability.

Color contrast can be useful to help people with visuospatial difficulties or poor eyesight. There should be enough contrast to be noticeable by aging eyes, but extremes of contrast can paradoxically cause difficulties with focus and discrimination.

I was told of one nursing home that significantly reduced their falls rate by simply putting wooden seats on the toilets. Their bathrooms had white toilets and white seats, against a backdrop of white tile floors and walls. People were missing the toilet seats and falling when they attempted to sit. The dark-colored seat greatly improved their ability to sit properly.

Adequate lighting will improve wayfinding and recognition, but proper attention to the right lighting for each area is also critical—high-quality ambient light for general navigation and targeted light for reading or handwork, not the other way around:

> Culture change specialist Nancy Fox was once asked to provide consultation for a large nursing home. While auditing the physical environment, she noted that the organization had taken pains to increase the intensity of light in the hallways; however, they used sconces with exposed bulbs. She showed me a photo she had taken looking down the hallway, and the camera image was almost totally washed out by glare from the bulbs. This would be a severe impediment to safe navigation for someone with aging eyes or cognitive limitations.

Careful attention to acoustics will also help produce an environment more conducive to relaxed, focused thought. At the same time, those with hearing loss should have hearing aids in place and working properly to maximize comprehension during conversation.

A Little-Recognized Barrier to Autonomy

Another lesson I learned in helping implement St. John's Green House homes was the way in which furniture—particularly beds—can have a powerful effect on autonomy. In exploring our own values during the design process, a common sentiment from the planning committee members was that people would want bigger, more comfortable beds than most nursing homes provide.

As I traveled to various conferences and trade shows, I would ask the vendors if they could make a full-size hospital bed. They all answered that slightly wider beds were available, but a true full-size bed was not being manufactured by anyone I met.

When leading the final design portion of our planning, Rebecca Priest decided to take matters into her own hands and brought a Tempur-Pedic®-style bed over from a residential mattress store for elders and staff to try. One man, living with quadriparesis, said, "Five minutes on this bed almost undoes five years of hell on my bed upstairs!" The response was overwhelmingly positive, and Priest purchased 20 beds for the homes.

The night that the first three residents moved into the home, they went to bed and slept until nearly 11:00 the next morning. One woman sheepishly said, "Oh, don't let me sleep so late!" A gentleman who had lived at our home for decades with a spinal dystrophy told me, "This is the first time in 27 years I've slept through the night."

It should be noted that these beds, while adjustable, do not elevate up and down. The staff members are using ceiling-mounted lifts, sheet pulls, and other ergonomic approaches for those who cannot easily sit or stand. This continues to be something of a burden for staff working at night regarding those who need extensive assistance while in bed; but they have been working hard to accommodate those frail elders because of the positive effect of the beds on their well-being. (St. John's has recently found a non-medical vendor who makes high–low queen-sized beds and is considering them for future use.)

In fact, the transformation of the people in the Green House homes led me to wonder how much our traditional hospital beds functionally disable people. A bad night's sleep can cause an increase in arthritic pain, reducing one's ability to walk and transfer the following day. It can also affect one's mood, increasing the chance of a verbal or physical outburst.

It seems that most homes are being penny-wise and pound-foolish when they buy small, uncomfortable hospital beds. How much do we add to our burden of care by not going the extra mile to provide a good night's sleep?

The "Dementia Village" Concept

I have been asked what I think about homes or communities that are entirely "dressed up" as in an earlier era, to approximate the time of the elders' more durable memories. I have very mixed feelings about this idea, beyond my objections to segregated living. On the positive side, it is important that older people are presented with a living environment that they can use successfully. Many newer appliances (even light switches and shower fixtures), in an effort to be modern and stylish, can be very "user-unfriendly." For those older people (with and without cognitive illness) who find it difficult to keep up with the lightning speed of technological advances, a simpler, scaled-down design is more likely to be useable. (My own efforts to help my mother purchase simple telephones or television sets has shown me how opaque these devices have become for someone who only wants to use them in the simplest manner possible.)

But being "user-friendly" is very different from creating a stage set from *Leave It to Beaver,* or some other 1950s-era television show, for several reasons. First of all, it assumes that everyone living there has the same attachment to that particular era. People's minds dwell on different times of their lives in a very unique way. Second, I do not subscribe to the belief that people simply journey back in time in a linear fashion, settling on some bygone year. I believe the majority become "time travelers," focusing at times on one era or another. (I have a few comments about "retrogenesis" coming up in Chapter 8.)

My third objection is that such a setting creates conflict and confusion when the modern world inevitably inserts itself; for example, the clothing and hairstyles of visitors or professional staff, the television shows, the cars driving by, or the 60-year-old man who walks in and says, "Hello, Mom." Like Fazio's definition of the evolving self (shared in Chapter 3), I believe people need a link to their past, but also a bridge to the present day and their evolving identity.

My last objection, most relevant to the domain of autonomy, is that many of the intrinsic changes associated with cognitive illness negate any purported benefit of those old-fashioned accoutrements. For example, if a person's problems with memory and executive function cause him to leave a lit stove unattended, it does not matter if the stove is a '50s-era Philco or an ultrasleek new LG range.

In summary, I think that if the people living in such communities are experiencing a high level of well-being, it is much more likely due to the way in which they are supported by their care partners and the overall deinstitutionalization of the living environment, rather than the retro furnishings or the segregation.

Control over Visitation

Gojikara Village in southern Japan also uses design to help enhance elder autonomy. In their assisted living apartment building, the elders live on the second floor; visitors enter on the ground floor and are greeted by nursing staff whose work area is a coffee bar. They are served coffee or tea and a call is placed to the elder, informing her that a visitor has arrived. Unlike a typical care home, where visitors may go to the living areas and knock on one's door unannounced, this arrangement puts the elder in charge of the visit. She can say, "Send them up," or "I'll be down in 10 minutes," or "Sorry, I'm not feeling well today." The choice is hers, and there is no risk of unwelcome intrusions.

Four Domains in Concert

Up to this point we have built a foundation for higher levels of self-actualization, even in people with significant cognitive limitations. There are three more domains to go. Before moving on to the important domain of meaning, I will share one last story, from Dr. Larry Lawhorne, the Chair of Geriatrics at Wright State University in Dayton, Ohio. This story illustrates that paying attention to the various well-being domains is also often helpful in defusing an acute situation of distress. In this story, the first four domains were combined effectively to resolve the crisis:

> Dr. Lawhorne was called by the staff at the nursing home where he was working because a gentleman had fallen to the floor. The staff had rushed over and determined that he was not injured, but he was resisting their attempts to help him stand, and they were at an impasse. Could he possibly come by and help?
> When he arrived on the scene, Lawhorne saw a figure lying supine on the floor with a number of staff standing over him,

shouting directions and trying to grab hold of his arms, as he swatted their hands away. The first thing he did was to ask everyone to move away from the man, thus giving him space and removing all of the figures looming over him (security).

Then, Lawhorne worked with the domains of identity and connectedness. His ongoing relationship with the man as his physician would help him to make a meaningful and trusted connection; but what was the best approach? Deciding to take connectedness literally to the next level, Lawhorne proceeded to lie down on the floor, eye-to-eye with the gentleman and said cheerfully, "Hey, Norm, how are you doing?"

Being at eye level and face-to-face, the man quickly recognized his doctor and greeted him enthusiastically. Then Lawhorne asked him, "Norm, do you know where we are right now?" The man asked, "Where?" and he replied, while patting the floor between them, "We're on the floor! What do you think we should do about that?" (autonomy).

The man considered the question and said, "I think we should get up." Lawhorne replied, "Me, too," and with his assistance, the man quickly rose to his feet and continued on his way. Crisis averted.

CHAPTER 7

Meaning

I don't take your words
Merely as words.
Far from it.
I listen
To what makes you talk—
Whatever that is—
And me listen.

—Shinkichi Takahashi

Those who have a "why" to live, can bear with almost any "how."

—Viktor Frankl

Being of use makes being in need easier.

—Wendy Lustbader

Meaning Defined

For me, "meaning" has, well, two meanings. Fox et al. (2005) define meaning as "significance; heart; hope; import; value; purpose; reflection; sacred." These facets of meaning are reflected, for example, in the work of Dan Buettner (2008), an explorer and researcher who has studied "blue zones" (areas of the world where people live and thrive to a very old age). Buettner observed elders on the island of Okinawa, Japan. Okinawans embrace the concept *ikigai*, which means "a reason to get up in the morning" and reflects their belief that each day must bring a sense of purpose. Buettner found a similar sense of purpose in each of the blue zones he has studied. The Fox et al. (2005) definition embodies this concept, as do many other models for well-being (e.g., the Murray Alzheimer Research and Education Program's [MAREP's] "making a difference"; Kitwood and Bredin's "sense of personal worth"; Nolan et al.'s "significance"; or Verity's "to feel needed and useful," each of which is mentioned in Chapter 2).

In addition to these facets of meaning, I also use this chapter to explore the "other meaning of meaning"; that is, how to interpret the messages that lie within people's words and actions. This is critical to understanding the needs of people living with dementia and is a vital component of enlightened communication skills. We touched on this in Chapter 4, but I like the idea of expanding the discussion here. So in various sections of this chapter, I will toggle between the concepts of "meaning–purpose" and "meaning–message."

We are now rising into rarefied air on the well-being pyramid. Identity and connectedness are essential in order to enhance security and autonomy. Security and autonomy, in turn, will promote opportunities for meaning and growth. And achieving these higher levels is a key to creating joy, even in the face of cognitive disability.

Since each level of well-being benefits from those below it, the higher levels are less concrete and more susceptible to the changes in those below. Accordingly, the ways in which these three remaining domains are expressed can have greater variation, both between different individuals and within one person over the course of time. The ways in which we enhance these domains are also less exact or prescriptive than the first four. Up to this point, we have devoted a lot of effort to breaking out of rigid thinking; it is important to continue to push ourselves even further because rigidity does not serve these higher domains any better than it does the domains of security and autonomy.

How Dementia Challenges Meaning

In this chapter, I have combined the discussion of intrinsic and extrinsic challenges because our own view of meaning is so closely tied to societal views around this concept. It is hard to understand the effects of cognitive disability without understanding how these larger issues shape them.

Intrinsic and Extrinsic Challenges

Industrialized society tends to attach meaning to doing, so any person who is unable to do as much will struggle to find meaning or recognition within these parameters. Meaning is most often recognized by society in relation to one's career, although child-rearing is often acknowledged as well. Of course, there are many other ways to engage meaningfully in the world, but they require more effort, because one has to generate his own internal source of validation and fulfillment.

> It is easier to live with the mandatory activity of work or child-rearing than to create voluntary purposes every day. (Lustbader, 1991, p. 2)

This is the dilemma facing those who are retired or unemployed, as well as those who live with chronic illness or disability. The change in cognitive abilities accompanying dementia compounds the problem, making it more difficult for a person to imagine and pursue a purposeful life. Societal stigmas regarding dementia reinforce the notion that one cannot be of use to others, and in the grief that usually accompanies the diagnosis, it becomes easy to embrace the notion that one's useful life is over.

As Shabahangi and Szymkiewicz (2008) remind us,

> We seem to take it for granted that a meaningful life is possible only when one is blessed with excellent memory and cognitive abilities. From this point of view, life makes little sense for the millions of Americans and countless others around the world afflicted with forgetfulness. (p. 12)

Each of the ways in which the first four well-being domains become eroded by stigma contributes to this loss of purpose. A societal view that the person is fading away, and the exclusion of such individuals that results, separates the person from any opportunity to engage in meaningful activity. Furthermore, creating meaning requires some risk—the risk to move outside one's comfort zone and accomplish something she has not done before. This is hard to achieve in a society preoccupied with downside risk. Finally, the view that people living with dementia can only receive care and have decisions made for them erodes autonomy, while meaning flows from the ability to make choices and give input into things that matter to oneself and others.

A desire to have a reason to get out of bed each morning does not end at the time of diagnosis, but the diagnosis of dementia often triggers an existential crisis (Power, 2010, p. 13). Central to such a crisis is the question, "What is my purpose in life, now that I have dementia?" If anything, people can become *more* preoccupied with finding meaning when they receive the news that they may have a progressive illness. Voris (Voris, Shabahangi, & Fox, 2009) recounted the hidden value of one of his closest friendships:

> What Bob brings to my life now is his belief that my life has value, that I've done things that are meaningful to him. Therefore, I am alive. And so I realize I will not die alone. (p. 16)

Frankl (1959) believed that an ability to find meaning in life, even a life with great suffering, is essential to human survival. If this is true, then helping those living with dementia to find and realize continued meaning in their lives is essential to their well-being, and possibly their longevity as well.

Needless to say, this requires us to challenge the stigmas that have defined dementia. In so doing we can imagine a different path that creates authentic partnerships and opportunities for the person to have an impact on the world around him. Unfortunately, even those of us who try to create meaning often do so from a standpoint that is too entrenched in the biomedical model of care.

The Shortcomings of Programmed Activities and "Therapeutic Recreation"

As should be evident by now, this book intends to challenge our current paradigms. Up to this point I have challenged many of the basic precepts of doctors, nurses, researchers, and those who work in segregated living areas. Now it is time to talk about our approach to recreation. So, at the outset, I will repeat my message that the professionals I have known and worked with are talented, creative, and passionate in their efforts to help those they serve. The aim of this discussion is not to invalidate these good people, but to challenge the *systems* that surround therapeutic recreation—the educational paradigm and the reductionist views it creates, as well as the system of reimbursement and regulation that perpetuates these views.

Our attempts to create meaning often fall short in the area of programmed activities, whether in the nursing home or in community day centers. There are several drawbacks to the way in which these are conceived and presented. Much of the activity in these settings falls into two categories: therapy that is aimed at deficits identified by standardized assessments, or entertainment (which is often passively experienced). Much of the assessment approach taught in professional school follows the deficit-based view of people living with dementia that characterizes the biomedical model. This is not to say that there is no role for rehabilitative therapy (or entertainment, for that matter) in people's lives. But the biomedical approach places such activity at the center and, therefore, fails to create meaning in a number of ways.

First, the assessments themselves are similar to those used to evaluate cognitive function; as such, they measure discrete tasks but do not capture integrative types of thinking. Activities that are directed by such tests may do little to improve one's overall cognitive function, and even less to create a meaningful experience. The approach is also often deficit based, rather than drawing on existing strengths. Furthermore, these activities often have a focus on biomedical outcomes, which gives a limited view of what a person needs to improve or maintain well-being. Eliopoulos (2010) observed that other dimensions of wellness (emotional, social, spiritual, and environmental) are often overlooked with this view. The result, according to Carson (2012), is that we "service the illness."

Bartlett and O'Connor (2010) expand upon the limitations of a biomedical approach to activities:

> In the dementia debate, "occupation" is usually quite narrowly defined and discussed only in terms of its psychosocial or therapeutic value. Moreover, the tendency in the field has been to create and speak of "artificial" environments. . . . Think, for example, about how outings for residents are often conceptualized as "meeting care needs" rather than as providing opportunities for people to access facilities in their local community that they are entitled to use—for example, museums, libraries, parks, adult education courses. (p. 42)

Another drawback of this approach is that it gives little or no consideration to the needs and desires of the individual and, therefore, is not person-directed. When many of the activities we provide are examined through the lens of our seven domains of well-being, they usually fall far short of the ideal. In addition, the reimbursement system for long-term care favors standardized "interventions," and so much of what would have been an organic leisure experience in the community becomes a packaged "therapy" that can be quantified and reimbursed as such, but often creates artificial forms of engagement.

Is this enough? Let us return once again to an examination of our own needs. I may spend some of my time engaged in activities designed to improve my health (exercise and diet) or improve skills that are lacking (reading a book on how to be better organized). But much of what occupies my time and interest outside of work is not based on deficits, but rather on meaning, growth, and joy.

I do not play the guitar, travel, or go for a hike to improve a physical disability, and I do not read, do crossword puzzles, or learn a foreign language to correct cognitive deficits. These are ways that I stimulate myself to experience the world in all its variety, become more than I am, and get in touch with an inner sense of peace or satisfaction. Are these goals only important to people with normal cognitive function? I think not.

In his own memoir of life with Alzheimer's, Robert Simpson (Simpson & Simpson, 1999) makes this plea: "I still want to be needed in some way. I would like you to talk things over with me, even if I can't respond well. I still need to hear 'I need you.' Even when I can't believe you do." (p. 38)

Unfortunately, activity that does not provide opportunities for meaning and growth is either entertainment or busy work, and this is not enough to create well-being. One of my favorite stories from Dr. Richard Taylor (2011) relates a visit he made to a nursing home where he was giving a talk:

> When speaking in nursing homes, Taylor likes to take time to visit some of the people who live there. One day he entered a dementia-specific living area and saw two women who would be described as having a moderate degree of cognitive disability.
>
> The women were busy with a pile of children's clothes that lay on the table in front of them; they were folding the clothes and placing them into a laundry basket. Taylor introduced himself and engaged them with pleasant conversation.
>
> After a few minutes, he asked the women if the clothes belonged to children of staff members or if there was a child care center in the building. One woman responded. "No, there are no children here."
>
> Pressing on, Taylor ventured, "Perhaps these are donations for the poor?" The woman looked at her companion and said, "Should we tell him?" Her friend nodded.

The woman turned back and said, "There are no children here. They bring us these clothes in a big pile, and we fold them and put them in the basket. Then they take them away somewhere, mess them up and bring them back, and we fold them again."

Taylor must have had a look of shock on his face; the other woman looked at him and hastened to add, "Yes, but it's better than a stick in the eye." He uses this story to implore nursing homes to give people something to do that is not simply "better than a stick in the eye."

In his presentations, Taylor often says that he needs "a purposeful and purpose-filled life"; in other words, days that are filled with meaning and that also create a pathway to greater fulfillment. He often asks residents of nursing homes, "Why did you get out of bed this morning?" and laments that most people he meets do not have a good answer.

From the standpoint of the physical environment, a living space that does not foster identity and connectedness will do little to add meaning to a person's life. Think about all of the things in your home or apartment that hold meaning for you. How much of that translates to the personal possessions, décor, relationships, or physical layout that you see in the typical skilled care or assisted living home?

Our second definition of "meaning"—the message behind one's words or actions—is invariably challenged by dementia for a number of reasons. In this case, the main intrinsic cause is not so much forgetfulness per se, but the other cognitive difficulties that can accompany the condition. These include word-finding difficulties and other challenges to speech, the tendency to move more fluidly through time, and (as Bryden suggested) the journey from a world of facts and memories to one of emotions and symbols. Each of these creates barriers to understanding and to being understood. We have touched upon this issue in previous chapters, and will do so in greater depth in the section on enhancing meaning at the end of this chapter.

Segregated Living and Meaning

The biomedical view of dementia is not limited to one type of environment, so a narrow or holistic view should not be more or less likely to occur in segregated environments. However, the philosophy behind segregation drives a more medicalized approach; so as we saw with autonomy, it is harder to rise above this type of thinking in such environments.

Because the living area is designed around dementia (or in some cases, a particular stage of dementia), this often dominates our view of the people who live there. The majority of segregated living areas that I have seen tend to focus their approach to leisure on a list of activities that are "appropriate for people living with dementia" (or, in some cases, "appropriate for people living with one stage of dementia").

Once again, this determination is made on the basis of standardized, deficit-based cognitive tests. But in addition to using scales that do not measure the person's full capabilities, this approach paints the residents of the living area with a broad brush, assuming that, based on these scores, certain activities will be most fulfilling for all.

There is nothing wrong with the idea that people need engagement on a level at which they can be successful. But if that is the only dimension we measure, then we are missing the other dimensions of wellness that Eliopoulos described earlier.

Suppose that Jim and Betty both achieve the same score on a Folstein Mini-Mental State Examination or Reisberg's Global Deterioration Scale? Does this mean that they should be engaged in the same activities? What if Jim is a married farmer with six children who loves baseball and hiking, and Betty is a single, retired teacher who loves jigsaw puzzles and mystery novels? Does the fact that they have the same cognitive score mean they will be equally served by the activities recommended for people at that level?

Once again, putting the disease before the activity squelches individualized care by assuming that everyone in a certain category has the same needs. Not only are many of the activities devoid of meaning for the individual, but such individuals may also be denied more meaningful or stimulating activities because their test scores do not recognize their ability to engage in more complex and integrative ways (e.g., sharing wisdom, providing emotional support to others, or traveling to a museum or concert hall to delve into works of art or music).

Lastly, many homes segregate people and provide level-specific activities based on the argument that it is easier for care partners to interact with and support people at one level of cognition. Again, this creates generalizations about what people need, and if a living area is designed primarily for staff efficiency or convenience, the chances are that individualized care is going to be lost.

With regard to my second definition of meaning, I have found that many people who work in such environments may have a greater knowledge of ways to respond to distress, but there are very few who truly understand how to "look past the words" and relate to the well-being needs that are symbolically expressed; as a result, the distress usually recurs, and medication use continues to be significant in these living areas as well.

In fact, a Cochrane Report (2012) was recently published regarding segregated living environments. This series of reports from Oxford University represents some of the most thorough literature reviews that can be found on various subjects. Their extensive review of the available research showed "no compelling evidence" that segregating people living with dementia produces better outcomes. Once again, one can point to individual organizations in both models of care that are excellent or inferior; but there is no evidence that the philosophy of segregation is superior.

Community-Based Living and Meaning

Erosion of meaning for those living in the community stems from the same views that permeate the nursing home. The societal view that people cannot learn and grow, that they cannot care for others or give meaningful input, and that they do not have a useful role in society also blinds family members to meaningful ways in which to engage their loved ones.

I will state a strong opinion here, and repeat it in the next chapter: Meaning and growth cannot be achieved in an environment that focuses simply on maintaining one's status quo or preventing decline. They can only flourish when our sights are set higher and we aim for something better than what we have today.

The activities that are provided in adult day programs and community senior centers fall prey to the same drawbacks as in the nursing home. And, as with the two women folding children's clothes, this is usually not lost on the participants. In fact, many of the expressions displayed by people during activities, such as pacing, calling out, or even striking out angrily at others, come as a reaction to the fact that the activity is devoid of meaning for them. One particular approach that can lead to such anger is an activity or interaction in which people are treated as children, as noted by Davis (1989):

> Watching some of the Alzheimer's day care centers featured on tele-
> vision gives me the "willies." I could never bear to be talked to and
> treated like a child at a summer camp. . . .
>
> I am repulsed by activity directors on cruise ships, much less some
> twenty-year-old trying to get me to play childish exercises to rock
> music. I am sure I would try to get back to my room and if stopped in
> this attempt I would become churlish and belligerent. If the insensi-
> tive director began to push or became condescending and began to
> pat my arm, I would probably explode with all the violence pent up in
> my six-foot-seven frame. If I were then restrained or tied in my chair,
> my fury would take me right out of my mind.
>
> Why? Is this the result of Alzheimer's disease? No, this is how I
> would react now in my best state of mind. . . . (p. 102)

Meaning is a function of many roles we inhabit in life—as a parent, a
spouse, a friend—as well as through our professions, our leisure time activities, or our faith. The emergence of dementia pulls the person away
from many of these roles, due to one's cognitive challenges and to one's
progressive exclusion by society. The result is an erosion of meaning,
of a reason to live.

But the knowledge of a progressive illness, even impending death,
does not remove the person's need for meaning. Voris (Voris et al.,
2009) found a renewed sense of purpose in his diagnosis:

> As it does for many human beings, the concept of death invokes both
> anxiety and resolve in me. Anxiety because death is the ultimate un-
> known, resolve because finitude can be the greatest benefactor of the
> life we lead on earth. (p. 21)

> Far from experiencing a time of fear and doubt, I feel privileged
> to be able to use my life to possibly make a contribution. No money—
> just life—used for all of us. Can it get any better than that? (p. 34)

Viewed in this light, enhancing meaning for those who live with dementia becomes of paramount importance because it gives individuals
a chance to come to terms with their mortality, knowing that they will
leave this earth having created a legacy and changed the world for the
better, even if in small ways. The key is to find and cultivate those small
ways, because once they stop, so does the will to go on.

Even when thinking about death, many people living with dementia see it as a way they can benefit others. In his 2003 memoir,
Larry Rose mused about wanting to donate his organs, and showed the

detail to which he thought about making sure that his wishes would be successfully carried out:

> Take all that is good and the junk that is left, just burn it and throw it to the wind. I will have already achieved a certain degree of immortality.
>
> I have made a videotape of what I want when the time comes for me to go. I have spelled it out exactly what I want [*sic*] and I don't want anyone taking part of it out of context. I don't want to do myself in because of the reasons just mentioned above. It might be a time before anyone finds me and by that time none of the organs would be of value to anyone. (p. 57)

One cannot separate the desire to give to others from a person's life, regardless of illness. In fact, many episodes of distress stem from people trying to act on this desire when there is no opportunity to do so. Enhancing meaning, therefore, not only creates a life worth living, it can also address the root cause of much distress.

Enhancing Meaning

I begin this last section with a discussion of how we can use personal, operational, and physical transformation to create a sense of purpose in life. I will then devote a separate section to understanding the message within one's words and actions.

Personal Transformation

We begin once again by looking inward and transforming our own understanding of what is meaningful for a person living with dementia. Meaning, like other aspects of well-being, must be driven at least in part by the individual. Meaning is created by activities that speak to one's own background, values, preferences, strengths, relationships, and spirituality. Any activity that is designed without taking these into account is likely to be too superficial to enhance this important domain, particularly for those who are struggling to find their own sense of purpose. Also, we need to remember that meaning is often created in states of *being* as well as doing. Much meaning arises in moments of solitude or quiet reflection, rather than activity. We must provide time and space for this as well.

In addition to enhancing meaning for the individual, Shabahangi and Szymkiewicz (2008) explain that dementia has a deeper meaning for all of us:

> In [our] book, we highlight a basic attitudinal shift: Dementia is our teacher. Rather than simply a disease, dementia has purpose and meaning. Rather than being people simply in need of our care, people who forget can teach us about life and living. Rather than a burden, people with dementia offer us an opportunity to deepen ourselves, to go deeper into our souls. (p. 12)

As with our other paired domains, we will see that meaning resonates closely with growth. The experience of caring for a person living with dementia creates meaning as well as growth for both the person and those who partner with her.

A key to creating meaningful moments is to remind ourselves that people living with dementia do learn, they do grow, and they are able to give care as well as receive it. Knowing the person is our key to finding how to enable these opportunities.

A certain amount of entertainment is enjoyable, but we also must consider activity that has a visible purpose. So folding laundry is not necessarily all bad, but there should be a point to it. Folding napkins to set on the table for dinner is very different from folding the same clothes over and over, simply to keep busy.

People must be able to relate activities to their personal lives and values, so it is important to develop facilitation skills that help care partners tie these in to each person's individual perspective. Such activities also need to provide space for participants to co-create the process, so that they remain in the flow and can express themselves fully.

Anne Basting's TimeSlips™ approach (discussed in *Dementia Beyond Drugs*, and at www.timeslips.org) is an excellent example of harnessing creative storytelling to co-create a shared narrative that produces creative engagement and expressive ability far beyond what standardized tests might predict.

To Feel, versus to Be

I propose another change in our language of support for people living with cognitive limitations, namely that we strike the word *feel* from our language in relation to activity or occupation. In other words, we need to stop saying that the goal of an activity is to help people to *feel* useful. The implication is that there may be an *appearance* of meaning, but that the activity may not be truly meaningful. This view enables subterfuge; such as having people fold towels, sort pencils, or engage in other busywork that does not serve a purpose or provide a tangible benefit for the person or those around her.

I suggest instead that we always ask, "What can the person do to *be* useful?" Do not assume that the person does not need to see tangible results, or have her work displayed and acknowledged in the life of the home.

The Power of the Moment

Another part of the interpersonal dynamic that is often overlooked is the power of being in the moment with a person living with dementia. Such people have an uncanny ability to focus on the present, perhaps in part because the past and future are less accessible. Meaningful connections are often best made when we can simply *be* with the person, remaining fully mindful and in the moment.

In such interactions, there is no need to perform, no right or wrong. The moment is what it is, and that space of unconditional acceptance often enables a person to express herself in ways that are impossible when tasks are being attended to. It also gives us the opportunity to notice things that we would normally overlook. These include small pleasures and connections, but also subtle clues to what aspects of the environment might be nurturing or eroding a person's sense of comfort and well-being.

Meaning and Failure

Finally, a sense of purpose is best acquired when one has a sense of *agency*; that is, the power to affect one's own destiny. Therefore, security and autonomy are important factors in enhancing meaning. Remember that risk has an upside as well as a downside. Meaning is often optimized when we are able to negotiate the downside successfully to enable the benefit to be realized:

> Psychologist Kort Nygard (2011) once told me a story that dramatically shifted my thinking about creating meaning. He was counseling a gentleman who had moved to assisted living and was feeling depressed. The man had laid floors for a living, but had to retire due to physical disability from arthritis, and then eventually was unable to care for himself at home.
>
> The gentleman was feeling as if he was no longer of use, and trying to find something meaningful in his present life.

> Nygard suggested that maybe the laundry staff could use some help with folding, but the man rejected that: "No, that's just 'busywork.' I need something *meaningful* to do!"
>
> Nygard then asked him, "Tell me then, what would be something to do that *you* would consider meaningful?" After a moment's consideration, the man replied, "I want a job to do where if I screw it up, something bad happens."

Now, a comment such as that would likely strike fear into the hearts of providers and regulators alike. But it made me think about what creates meaning in the work we pursue. I realized that meaning comes from the possibility of failure—of downside risk. If we pursued a task that had no possibility of failure, then there would be no meaning in completing it successfully. Meaning (as well as growth and joy) results from knowing that we accomplished something that may have failed, but did not.

The lesson here is that failure-free activities are usually devoid of meaning. Our emphasis on surplus safety often carries over to the types of activities that are provided to people living with dementia. Even a young child will become bored with a game if you let him win all the time. Therefore, in facilitating activities, it is the wrong question to ask, "How can we make this activity failure-free for the participants?" A better question is, "How can we facilitate an activity where people can succeed, but where they can also (safely) fail from time to time?" (Once again, there is a correlate in the domain of growth that will be discussed in Chapter 8.)

Operational Transformation

There are many ways in which we can shift our approach to care and support in order to create opportunities for meaningful engagement for people in all living environments. The following are a few important examples to consider.

Rituals

One of the most important ways in which we can transform operations to enhance meaning is through the creation or restoration of important rituals. One of the primary ways in which institutional living erodes meaning is by turning important rituals (e.g., mealtime, holidays, birthdays, death) into sterile routines. (I discuss this process in depth in Chapter 7 of *Dementia Beyond Drugs*.)

Routines involve the completion of tasks, but usually without underlying meaning or significance for the individuals involved. Rituals create meaning in a variety of ways—by attaching memories, relationships, traditions, individuality, inclusion, culture, and often spirituality to the activity. Rituals are particularly crucial for those who are forgetful, helping to sustain durable memories and attaching purpose to a daily life that often seems to hold none.

Rituals have the following components:

- a defined beginning or welcoming of those who participate
- engagement and inclusion of all in the activity
- tie-in to personal histories, traditions, and values
- flexibility to accommodate different abilities
- central importance of relationship in proceeding through the activity
- an experience that is more important than the result
- a closing and appreciation for those who attended

In various living environments, it is worth taking the time to look at each activity of the day and decide if it can be "ritualized" by enhancing these components. Any activity, from getting up in the morning to going to bed at night and everything in between, can be transformed into a more meaningful experience. In the nursing home or assisted living environment, there should be a combination of preserving old rituals and creating new ones to help the person find meaning within his current living space. In fact, even when someone is living at home, a combination of old and new rituals needs to be considered, to accommodate the changing needs and abilities of the person living with dementia.

Shanks's approach to getting her husband ready for the bath described in Chapter 6 is a good example of the establishment of a new ritual in one's home. St. John's Home in Rochester, New York, has created many rituals to help people create meaning and memory in a new living environment. One is the annual Water War, in which two neighborhoods and a diverse group of employees meet in the courtyard on a warm summer day, dress in bathing suits or clothing protectors, and soak each other with water pistols, water balloons, and spray bottles.

Another ritual is the annual Illumination of Love, in which the auxiliary committee solicits donations for the decoration of a tree in December for the various holidays. Each $5 donation represents one white light on the tree, each of which is dedicated to a special person, past or present, and the decorating is capped off with a gala Sunday evening lighting ceremony. Each of these rituals creates a sense of belonging for those who may feel displaced from the lives that they had previously known, and shows that the way forward, while often difficult, is not traveled alone.

Living and Celebrating Life through Leisure

Because of the shortcomings of the biomedical view of programmed activities, another good place to start is one that rethinks this process. DuPuis, Whyte, and Carson (2012) outline a new vision for creating a different approach to meaning, applicable to all living environments. Echoing the sentiments expressed by Bartlett and O'Conner earlier in the chapter, they seek to move beyond the narrow view of recreation as a series of activities focused on therapeutic goals to the concept of a leisure *experience*. This concept was developed as a practical application of the *authentic partnerships* approach mentioned in Chapter 2 (DuPuis, Gillies, Carson, et al. 2012). The researchers worked in partnership with people living with dementia, family members, and professionals to create a new recreation resource guide.

The shift to a leisure experience helps overcome two limitations of the traditional approach: (1) it moves beyond the narrow biomedical goal of activities, and (2) it broadens our view of recreation to incorporate both doing and being. The authors cite yet another shift:

> Rather than developing an assessment tool *for* people with dementia, researchers, professionals and family members are partnering directly *with* people with dementia to develop an assessment tool and evaluation approach that is most relevant to them as well as to better support people with dementia in continuing to thrive and live a quality life. (DuPuis, Gillies, Carson, et al., 2012, p. 225)

Implicit in this quote is the fact that the leisure experience, like well-being, is a multifaceted concept that requires a knowledge of the individual to achieve. It was through this working group (a collaborative with the Murray Alzheimer Research and Education Program) that their seven most valued dimensions of *being me, being with, finding balance, seeking freedom, making a difference, growing and developing,* and *having fun* were identified.

The authors quote Pedlar, Hornbrook, and Haasen (2001), who stated that "leisure experience involves spontaneity and internal motivation" (p. 16), implying that the more traditionally applied approaches, in trying to maximize efficiency and consistency, restrict individual choice. In fact, Sylvester (1987) calls leisure "the celebration of freedom at its crowning point" (p. 81).

The assessment, adapted from Pedlar et al. (2001, p. 27) and remarkably simple and straightforward, consists of five questions:

1. What do you enjoy? (past and present leisure interests)

2. What about that do you enjoy? (characteristics of pursuits that are enjoyed)

3. Recently, what has brought enjoyment and happiness to your day? (current leisure status)

4. What is stopping you from enjoying _____ (or some of these activities)? (barriers)

5. Is there something you have always wanted to do? (dreams)

These questions are simple, and their open-ended nature lends to highly individualized responses, keeping the person's desires and needs at the center of the assessment.

Does this approach negate the value of therapeutic recreation specialists? Not at all, but it shifts their role in long-term living environments. Instead of assessing and prescribing through the traditional approach, these specialists learn new ways of partnering with people living with dementia and their families to create a leisure experience rich with individual meaning. Specific therapies to target areas of need can continue to be used, but they do not replace leisure as the only approach to daily occupation. Furthermore, this approach may increase the professional's openness to soliciting the person's input into the more traditional therapeutic activities as well.

Lastly, the professional can act as a resource for other care partners, helping them develop their skills in facilitating leisure experiences throughout the day. In this manner leisure can truly enjoy the spontaneity that it requires, matching the ebb and flow of the individual's daily rhythm, rather than waiting for a predesignated day and time for engagement. This, in turn, will create meaning for the individual and foster opportunities for growth.

Volunteering and Mentoring Opportunities

One important way to create meaning and fight the stigmas of dementia is to enlist people living with cognitive change in activities in which they can continue to share their wisdom and skills to the benefit of others. Such opportunities can be created in all living environments, with the proper support.

In the community, a volunteer opportunity serves to combat the existential crisis felt by people who are diagnosed with dementia by reassuring them that their life is not over simply because of their illness. Volunteer opportunities offer a pathway to meaning for many who might feel otherwise marginalized, including people without dementia who are coming to terms with a shift in their societal role after retirement.

In 2011, I shared a speakers' forum with Tara Stringfellow of Alzheimer's Australia, Western Australia (AAWA). Stringfellow helped spearhead a program sponsored by AAWA to connect community residents living with early-stage Alzheimer's with volunteer opportunities in their community. This program has successfully created meaningful roles for people whom society might otherwise marginalize, and areas of need in the community benefit as well.

I have met many people in my travels who include family members living with dementia in their community work. A person may bring a spouse to a nursing home where she volunteers, to assist with a food drive or other charitable work. Many people who serve on the board of local Alzheimer's support chapters bring a family member to meetings and conferences. Some conferences, such as the Edna Gates Conference in Troy, Michigan, and A Changing Melody in Ontario, Canada, had people living with dementia on their planning boards and giving presentations. (Unfortunately, the Edna Gates Conference is currently inactive and there are few others like these in operation.)

Volunteerism is not restricted to people living in the community. Mission View Health Center, a nursing home in San Luis Obispo, California, engaged its elders in producing handmade soaps, which they sold at a local market to raise money for local charities. As the process evolved, their sights continued to rise. They began taking donations to the local charities, so that the elders could see the beneficiaries of their charity. Other charitable projects have resulted, and they became the first home in the nation to form a resident-based nonprofit organization, Helping Hands, to support their work.

People living with dementia are included on the volunteer projects to the best of their ability. Residents of Mission View have even received training as hospice volunteers in order to help their neighbors at the end of life.

One of the benefits of small house models such as the Green House® Project is that maintenance of the home becomes a central part of daily life. Therefore, the elders who live there can be engaged in activities that have a direct and visible effect on life in the home. They can plan meals, accompany staff on shopping trips, set tables, and prepare food as able. They also attend household meetings to give input into the weekly schedules and any issues that arise regarding life in the home. While traditional homes have a representative "Resident Council," the scale and locality of this model ensure that all have an important voice in daily life.

Skilled care partners who are sensitive to people's need for meaning can create small meaningful experiences, even for those with greater degrees of disability. Camp (2012) described a gentleman at one nursing home who loved to sing but forgot the words to all but a few romantic ballads. His frustration forced him to withdraw from musical activities, but an alert activity professional used a strength-based approach to re-engage him:

> She found out which ballads he could remember, and asked him if he would help her with a social event that involved a dinner for residents and their families. She wrote down the names of the songs that he could remember on a tablet. His job during the dinner was to go to different tables and ask people if they would like to hear a song. If they said yes, he would show them the list of songs that he knew and ask them which one they would like him to sing. In this way, he demonstrated his remaining abilities and the staff member helped him circumvent his deficits. This allowed him to fulfill a meaningful and entertaining social role. (p. 29)

Camp's book shares many such examples, including taking elders who had withdrawn from traditional activities and engaging them in the process of teaching Montessori-based activities to young children:

> The transformation in these older adults was truly amazing. I remember seeing men literally wake up so that they could teach children how to use a screwdriver and a socket wrench. I remember hearing them say, "Lefty—loosey; righty—tighty. Now you say it." Residents would teach children how to fold/hang their clothing, set a place at the table, sound out words, etc. Working with children was the highlight of their day. (p. 72)

As you can see, these examples show how the seven domains of well-being feed into each other and how the lines between them become blurred. There are elements of all of the domains we have discussed in the preceding two examples, and one can also see that the upcoming domains of growth and joy are represented as well. One can always identify a strong approach to engagement because it feeds so many domains of well-being simultaneously.

In fact, these stories show the close resonance between meaning and growth. When we engage in activities that are meaningful to us, it enables our continued growth, in spite of our physical or cognitive limitations. Both stories tell of people who were frustrated and withdrawn but who became re-energized, thereby benefiting themselves as well as those around them. They became teachers, care partners, mentors, bringers of joy—something to which we all aspire.

By Us, For Us

One way in which MAREP has used the authentic partnership approach with great success is the publication of their *By Us For Us*© guides. These booklets share experiences and advice for those who have been diagnosed with dementia and their loved ones, and were written by community members who live with dementia along with their care partners. The idea came from Brenda Hounam, who was diagnosed with Alzheimer's at age 53. She felt that she needed more information on her illness, especially from the perspective of those who shared her experience. Partnering with the University of Waterloo, Brenda and MAREP have seen the release of 10 different guides, covering such topics as enhancing communication, living and transforming with loss and grief, and managing triggers.

The U.S. Alzheimer's Association estimates that, on average, someone develops diagnosable symptoms every 67 seconds. When such a large number of people are confronted with this diagnosis, they can quickly succumb to the burdens of grief and stigma long before cognitive capacity is seriously diminished. What better way is there to start taking control and gaining the wisdom to engage proactively with your life and loved ones than with a resource such as the *By Us For Us*© guides?

There are many more ways that people living with cognitive disability can create meaning in all types of communities. I hope that these examples will show the variety of ways in which we can envision and operationalize pathways to a meaningful life for all. In the next chapter, we will revisit some of these concepts, tying them in with growth and self-actualization.

One last caution, however: Well-being cannot be actualized in people living with dementia if well-being is not experienced by their care partners as well. This is applicable to all seven domains, but the domain of meaning is a particularly good place to revisit the issue. In the community, how does society value those who are providing care to a loved one? In the nursing home, what kind of meaning and respect is afforded those who do this work for a living, largely using their time and effort to help those to whom they have no family ties?

Dr. Patrick Fox (Voris, Shabahangi, & Fox, 2009) summed up this quandary:

> It's an interesting fact that many of the things that are the most meaningful are the ones that are less valued from the standpoint of the overarching economy and status systems of the society. Caregiving is an example of that. (p. 33)

Once again, using the framework of well-being in caring for those who live with dementia teaches us the importance of the larger issue of creating well-being for their partners in care. This in turn has critical lessons for how we need to exist as a society, especially one in which our frail and elder population will dramatically increase in the years to come (see Chapter 11).

Physical Transformation

How do we create meaning in our physical design? Much of it flows from designing for the first four well-being domains we discussed: personalizing aspects of the living area, engaging people in relating to those aspects in a personal way, creating familiarity and comfort, and enabling people to have important input into how the environment is designed.

Furthermore, bringing these concepts together around the topic of meaning should make it clear that physical transformation alone will not create a meaningful environment unless we also use our operations to connect people to it in meaningful ways. For example, a personalized, comfortable, attractive dining room will have much more meaning if the inclusion of all parties and the preservation of important rituals around the dining experience are honored.

Kiyota (personal communication, November 4, 2013) adds that another operational aspect of meaning involves engaging family members in helping with the physical environment. There is often a lot of guilt associated with moving a loved one to a care home. By helping their family members to create meaning in the new living space, the family also finds the meaning (and connectedness) that helps them come to terms with this transition.

The Other Side of Meaning

As promised, I will now address the other definition of "meaning" described earlier—the message that lies within our words and actions. I have touched on this topic in earlier chapters and in my first book, and we can gain a bit more insight by understanding the perspective of the person and looking through the lens of well-being.

The first important step is to understand and accept that words and actions *do* have meaning, even if this is not apparent to us at the outset. Earlier, we discussed reframing "confusion" as a brain actively trying to understand, problem-solve, and communicate needs through newly damaged connections. Henderson (1998) puts it this way:

> People with Alzheimer's do actually think—they may not think the same sorts of things that normal people think, but they do think. They wonder how things happen, why things happen the way they are, and it's a mystery. (p. 21)

So why is it such a mystery? There are many factors. People with changing cognitive abilities receive information differently and process it differently. They may have word-finding difficulties that hamper their responses or attempts to communicate. They may be more fluid in time than we are. They are grieving and struggling with the erosion of all of these aspects of well-being. They often live in artificial environments that do not offer guidance or that contain confusing messages.

And on top of all of this, they think less on the level of memories and facts and more on the level of emotions and symbolism. This can be seen as compensation for lost cognitive skills, but it also reveals a deeper, even richer and more meaningful way of seeing the world around us—one that is often invisible to those of us whose thoughts are still bound by the rules of memory, logic, and linear time.

What happens when a person does not follow the "rules" of cognition? In our biomedical model, the result is pathology. But to understand the meaning behind the words and actions of those who do not follow these rules, we also need to free ourselves of the judgment of right and wrong, healthy and diseased, and see the world in a more neutral light.

> This shift of attitude . . . requires foremost a curiosity, an openness to all that is. An attitude of *not-knowing* allows that which manifests itself in front of or within us to present itself in the way it *is*, not the way we already know it. (Shabahangi & Szymkiewicz, 2008, p. 13)

Here is where both aspects of meaning come together. What appears confused, even delusional, to us may be the sign of a person trying to attach meaning (purpose) to her current experience. What we view as pathology may actually be a deeper awareness of levels of meaning than we ourselves possess!

Shabahangi and Szymkiewicz (2008) explore the ramifications of this in an altogether different, and very challenging, way by explaining the drawback of living in the "random" universe our perspective reflects:

> In such a universe, we do not strive for meaning, but rather to manage the suffering that occurs when meaning eludes us. That is, symptom removal or alleviation is the final goal. After the symptom is removed, we don't need to understand it anymore. In a random universe, we distinguish between good and bad, right and wrong, acceptable and unacceptable.
>
> Those who believe in a meaningful universe suffer, too, but their suffering gives rise to a desire to understand the meaning of that suffering, to delve more deeply into the reason and purpose of the events that occur in our and other people's lives. . . . (p. 13)

> People with forgetfulness go to their inner world more often and in a more profound way than we do. They are afraid of losing contact with everyday reality, but they are also searching for something important in their own inner world. . . . As they try to find the meaning of their experience, they use movement, sounds, repeated phrases, or stories to try to communicate with us. (p. 32)

Our charge, therefore, is to suspend judgment and try to understand. And if we cannot understand, at least to accept that what we do not understand has meaning on some level and has a legitimate place in the world of experience and expression. Only when we free ourselves of such judgments can we be open to a deeper understanding. Shabahangi and Szymkiewicz (2008) use the term *consensus reality* to refer to that which we accept as normal. The implication is that there are other realities, and even if we do not inhabit them, we need to appreciate their existence. Which brings us right back to the experiential definition of dementia and the important mindset it creates.

Now that I have hopelessly contaminated your orderly, scientific view of dementia, let us take advantage of our confusion and use it to look into the "confusion" of others, with new eyes. Cathie Borrie (2010) recalled a conversation with her mother, living with Alzheimer's, who had addressed her by her brother's name. Borrie asked, "Do you know who I am, Mum?" to which her mother replied, "*Do you?*" (p. 163).

The Logic behind Illogical Expressions

When we get hung up on the superficial meaning of words, they can appear illogical. It is only through understanding how they fulfill others' needs that we can see past this. Camp (2012) shares a story of a woman who repeatedly called out the name of her daughter, Jamie, after awakening from her nap each day:

> Staff members would come in and tell her, "Jamie's not here. What do you need?" This was a highly irritating and frustrating occurrence, and it took place each day . . . One day, a rehabilitation therapist came into the woman's room and said to the resident, "Why do you yell out your daughter's name every day when you wake up?" The woman looked up at the therapist and calmly said, "When I wake up, I need a nurse to help me. I never know who the nurse is going to be. But if I yell for my daughter, SOMEONE always comes." (pp. 23–24)

It can be very enlightening to simply ask "why," and yet when we are fixated on the paradigm of confusion, we never think that there might be an internal logic to a person's actions. And we never think about how our actions and responses may actually reinforce those expressions.

Nygard (2012) tells the story of a man living in a nursing home who kept coming into the kitchen area in the evening. The staff would congregate there, and he was likely drawn by the sound and looking for company. But the kitchen was considered "off limits" to the residents of the home. In an effort to redirect him, the staff would give him a cookie to go back to his room. Can you guess what effect this had? It was a perfect study in conditioned response—he returned even more enthusiastically on subsequent evenings. Who wouldn't?

Sometimes, the visual image a person sees, combined with past memories, can cause a reaction that looks confused or agitated. This can stem from being raised in a time when certain images carried other connotations, leading to a different interpretation than we might expect.

At St. John's Green House homes there is a spa room in each home that has a whirlpool tub for those who might prefer a bath to a shower. One woman who desired a bath was brought to the room with the tub already full and the whirlpool jets running. She immediately became upset and would not let the staff lift her into the tub. As the staff members further explored her reaction, she expressed the fear that she would be "boiled alive," as the whirlpool bath conjured up the image of a pot boiling on the stove. The water, steamy and bubbling, looked like it was far too hot for a bath. This reflected the woman's attachment to an era when Jacuzzi tubs were not commonly seen in America.

Lastly, sometimes the meaning is simpler than we expect. Pearce (2007) shares the story of a visit to a woman living with dementia and congestive heart failure who was felt to be very close to death. Although she had difficulty finding words, she managed to share with Pearce that she had seen her (deceased) husband, who told her they would soon go away together. Pearce told the woman how much she had enjoyed her visits, and that she would miss her. After a moment of reflective silence, the woman told her, "I have to go." Pearce told her that it was okay to let go, to join her husband, but the woman shook her head and seemed upset and unable to speak. Pearce offered to sit with her, and the woman nodded. Pearce continued to talk to her about her family, her faith, her future. "She merely shook her head and shrugged at everything I said. Very gradually she began to look more frustrated and even sadder. She eventually said very softly, very discreetly, and with much embarrassment, 'Pee'" (p. 232).

Thinking and acting in her usual role as a hospice worker, Pearce had missed one of the most common meanings of the expression, "I have to go." She apologized and called a staff member to assist her. And an hour later, much more comfortable and at peace, the woman finally made her journey.

Beyond the Words

We have discussed the extraordinary sensitivity to nonverbal signals that people living with dementia often possess. We often suppress these deeper intuitions in going about our daily activities; but when higher-level processes disappear or become less dominant, this deeper level of knowledge is released. Is this merely a process of "degeneration?" You be the judge:

> The homes of SentryCare in Mississippi have engaged elders in a variety of ways, not the least of which is including them in group interviews of prospective staff members. They have occasionally included people living with dementia in this process.
>
> On one such interview, a woman living with dementia joined a group of staff members. When the interview was over and the applicant left the room, they went around the table to share their thoughts. Each person in turn voiced approval of the applicant, until they came to the woman with dementia.
>
> "I wouldn't hire her," she flatly announced to the group. Perplexed, they asked for her reasoning. The woman proceeded to point out the applicant's nonverbal signals, of which she had been acutely aware. The woman said all the right words, but her posture, tone of voice, lack of eye contact, and other body language belied her answers. She struck the woman as being an expert in "interviewing," but completely insincere.
>
> The group was somewhat chastened by her insights. The applicant was not hired.

As this story illustrates, the amplification of nonverbal understanding is not simply a loss of higher function, but a sharpening of intuitive skills. In the contemporary business parlance, one could say that people with dementia often increase their "EQ." So, as noted in *Dementia Beyond Drugs*, a person who states, "They don't like me here," might be viewed as suspicious or paranoid, but could actually be experiencing very real body language from her care partners; body language that may represent feelings as varied as frustration, preoccupation, judgment, or disengagement, but that manifests as negative energy directed toward the person.

In this case, the body language may be entirely unintentional, but the effect is the same, and we may receive a negative reaction in return. Then we wonder why the person did not respond positively to our kind words, not realizing that our nonverbal language was drowning them out.

Our own preoccupation with other concerns can affect our ability to be open and present with the person, which can then interfere with the person's ability to focus and feel secure. Like all people who care for a person living with dementia, Borrie (2010) had to deal with her own grief, frustration, and the demands placed on her personal life. During one visit, an exchange about her mother's will shows how the underlying emotions raised each person's level of anxiety:

> I show her a copy of the will.
> *That's not mine.*
> "Yes it is, see where you've signed it?"
> *That's not my signature.*
> "Oh, I'm all mixed up, Mum. Let's just change the subject, it's getting irritating."
> *It was from the word go.*
> "Would you like a cup of tea?"
> *Oh how lovely. Where is my will? Did you sign this one?*
> "No! Oh gee . . . I think I'll go home now. . . . It's just too crazy here today."
> *It wasn't before you got here.* (pp. 86–87)

This is a beautiful example of both the frustration and humor that often lie behind such conversations. But it is also worth noting the nonverbal aspect of the exchange. Borrie was clearly finding the conversation "irritating," and it showed. So when she tried to divert her mother with a cup of tea, her body language was holding her mother in the anxious feeling of needing a will. Her increased anxiety caused her to fixate further, which in turn brought Borrie's frustration to the breaking point. Her final comment is all too telling—sometimes our body language creates or perpetuates the "craziness" for the person with dementia, thus heightening her anxiety and creating a vicious cycle.

Note the essential mismatch between Borrie, fixed in the factual reality of having a duly signed will, and her mother, who was expressing deeper emotional concerns about her family's financial security by repeatedly asking about the will. This is why repeated reassurances about the "fact" of her signature did not serve to calm her mother. (More on this mismatch in a moment.)

Getting Past the Word Choices

Often we get so hung up on the correctness of word choices that we miss the deeper meaning being expressed. When people have difficulty finding words and live in a world that places so much emphasis on conversation, they do the best they can to take part. But words often become interchanged or substituted with other words that may have a similar sound, a similar meaning, or a symbolic meaning or that may perhaps express a visual image that mirrors the emotion being expressed.

In one encounter with her mother, Borrie (2010) noted that she appeared somewhat sad. In her beautiful manner of asking open-ended questions that enable free expression, Borrie asked her mother, "What does sorrow look like?" Her mother responded, "It's a form of sadness brought on by a gray and heavy day. I've reached the ultimate of the intimate and that's the end of it" (pp. 135–136).

Note how the words switch to appropriate images of sorrow, and how the words at the end, while nonsensical on the surface, point to questions of identity, connection, and mortality. And note the poetry, the internal rhythm and rhyme: *ultimate, intimate, end of it.*

Shabahangi and Szymkiewicz (2008) also see the creativity and meaning behind those whose sense of time seems jumbled:

> Old people often use an object like a wedding ring to symbolize something from the past.
>
> A person in present time, like yourself, can represent a mother or sister.
>
> When old people combine one thought with another, they are often very poetic. (p. 61)

Furthermore, they remind us that "the purpose of remembering and reconstructing the past and telling stories is to find the meaning in life's journey" (p. 96).

Logic versus Symbolism

Now let us expand further on Christine Bryden's view of the journey from a world of facts and logic to one of emotions and symbolism. This is where we most need to let go of our present reality and enter that of the person living with dementia, understanding it on the deeper plane of well-being. We then see the comments, not for the accuracy of the words, but as a symbolic need to repair one or more aspects of well-being.

The earlier conversation about the will could be related to an erosion of security (and possibly autonomy as well). A comment about needing to fetch one's children from school could indicate a need to nurture and give care to others, a lost sense of security from displacement, or the reawakening of part of one's identity due to sights and sounds around a certain time of day. The statement "I want to go home" could indicate losses in all seven domains, or perhaps a desire to leave this life entirely. But until we identify, validate, and address the need being expressed, we will continue to miss the point.

Understanding this concept of thinking more on the level of emotions and symbols can lead to dramatic insights:

> I discussed this concept at a talk I gave in Alaska at the Juneau Pioneers' Home in 2012. A potluck supper and a social hour followed my late afternoon presentation to staff, elders, and families. After dinner, the daughter of a woman who had recently moved to the home approached me and thanked me for sharing this idea. "It helped me solve a problem I've been having with my mother," she told me. I asked her to elaborate.
>
> She explained that her mother had only arrived a few weeks before, and that she usually visited in the evenings after work. When the time came to say "good night," her mother would invariably ask, "But where are you going to sleep?" Her daughter's answer was always the same: "At home, of course."
>
> This response, while factual, led to her mother becoming sad, missing her home and family, and wanting to leave. It had become such an emotional event that her daughter was considering decreasing the frequency of her visits because it was so difficult to disengage.
>
> After thinking about her mother's question more in relation to emotion and symbolism, the daughter saw things on a different level. "She wasn't asking me literally where I was going to sleep. She was expressing that she is my mother and that she cares about my happiness, safety, and well-being.
>
> "So tonight after dinner, when I took her back to her room, she asked me the same question. This time, I said, 'Oh Mom, I have the most wonderful bed to sleep in tonight. I have a good book and I am going to curl up with a cup of tea and have a lovely evening.' And she smiled at me and said, 'Good night,' and I walked out the door."

Such needs will continue to be expressed until we understand and respond to them. This explains why the woman's question was so persistent, night after night, and why it resolved so dramatically when the underlying symbolism was understood.

During an education session earlier in the day, a staff member at the same home remarked that her family often tells her sister that she repeats herself. Her sister usually replies, "That's right; and I am going to continue to repeat myself until you listen!"

Symbolic word choices are another way in which people express themselves. Wong (2009) recounts a conversation with his mother after a shopping trip:

> "I was doing shopping in the child's car," she said, quite pleased with her "purchases."
>
> . . . A 92-year-old woman recounting a ride in a child's car? Then it struck me—she had personalised the wheelchair, humanising cold metal with humour, squeezing freedom out of immobility, turning a routine lunch trip into a joyride. She was light-heartedly mocking her state, an adult having to sit in a child's car. (pp. 139–140)

It is important not to simply discount what sounds like improper word choices. The substitutions may sound random, but they may be quite telling.

"Hallucinations" and "Delusions"

In *Dementia Beyond Drugs*, I devote an entire chapter to this subject, looking at the many ways in which the misperceptions of dementia can be improperly labeled as psychotic symptoms. I further expand upon this here, given that my views are outside of the mainstream of medical thinking.

Let me begin with an assertion I have made before—one that contradicts many textbooks on the subject, but reflects the reality of my more than 25 years in practice (which are enhanced by looking through an experiential lens): I believe that hallucinations and delusions in people living with dementia are more often than not improperly diagnosed.

There are several problems with these two labels. First, most of what we observe does not fit the psychiatric definitions of these disorders. We hear something that sounds bizarre to us, so we rush to label it as a psychotic symptom, when actually it is often a misperception of the environment by a person with shifting cognitive pathways. If a person lives in a home where strangers come and go without boundaries and if she forgets where she placed her purse, it is reasonable to conclude that someone may have come into her room and stolen it. That is not a delusion.

Second, many of the actions people exhibit represent their attempts to engage with the world by working around the gaps left by damaged brain connections. A person with a paralyzed left arm would look quite strange to the casual observer if he were trying to operate an old-fashioned can opener by using his one working arm and other parts of his body to stabilize the can. But that may be the only way he can compensate for his loss of function, so it makes the most sense to him. Many "delusions" reflect a similar process of compensation for lost information.

Another example of changing perception in a person with neurological damage might be the "phantom pain" caused by severed nerves from an amputated limb. That is not a hallucination and would not respond to antipsychotic medications.

Third, the brain chemistry of dementia is different from that of schizophrenia. In schizophrenia there appears to be heightened activity of the chemical dopamine. Although the genesis of delusions is probably not that simplistic, the use of a drug that blocks dopamine activity (as antipsychotics do) has some rationale here. But in the various forms of dementia, dopamine levels are decreased, or else remain normal. So it is easy to see why a dopamine blocker would not have the same effect. In fact, it is astounding that people who hold to a biomedical view of dementia would cling to drugs that have little biochemical basis for effectiveness.

Fourth, hallucinations, when they truly occur, are often not due to the dementia itself. In schizophrenia, hallucinations are almost always auditory and often involve hearing accusatory voices and feelings of others controlling one's thoughts. This is not the rule in dementia, where most perceptual problems are visual. Visual hallucinations are a hallmark of drug toxicity or withdrawal, and it is often the pills, not the dementia, that are the cause.

Drugs that block acetylcholine are known to be problematic in most forms of dementia, in addition to pills that raise dopamine levels, such as anti-Parkinson medications. But it is interesting to note that an increase of acetylcholine can also sometimes cause hallucinations because the chemical works differently in different areas of the brain. I find it fascinating that there are no studies to address this, because virtually everyone with a diagnosis of dementia these days is given one or more prescriptions for drugs that increase acetylcholine in the brain (e.g., donepezil or memantine). When we think someone is hallucinating, it never occurs to us that the cause may be their "Alzheimer's pill."

Neurologist Peter Whitehouse (Whitehouse & George, 2008) experimented with taking donepezil back in 2002 to test its effects on his own concentration. Unfortunately, he had to discontinue the medication after several days because of gastrointestinal upset, but while taking the pills he noted "some quite entertaining but disturbing dreams, that likely were by-products of the drug." The experience made him wonder if his patients had similar effects, "but, because of their dementia, lack the ability to articulate their discomfort" (p. 118). Furthermore, when they *can* be articulated, how many such symptoms will be considered hallucinations and attributed to their dementia?

What about the case of Lewy body dementia? This form of dementia affects the visual center of the brain as well as other areas, and bizarre visual sights are often noted. These may take the shape of a well-formed hallucination. But another confounding problem is that almost all such people have also been put on anti-Parkinson medications for their rigidity (even though these drugs work very poorly in this condition), and it may often be those pills that are contributing to the hallucinations. In response, many doctors simply add an antipsychotic, rather than decreasing or stopping the other pill. This is doubly harmful, because people with Lewy body dementia are extremely sensitive to the side effects of antipsychotics.

Many of the visual experiences of such people can be compensated for without resorting to antipsychotic pills. And, once again, these visual phenomena appear to be largely due to changes in the vision center of the brain, rather than a traditional mechanism of psychosis, and, therefore are much less likely to respond to antipsychotic drugs. There appears to be decreased circulation to the visual center of the brain, which may be an important cause of these visual phenomena; in fact, some studies suggest that the use of cholinergic drugs (e.g., donepezil) may increase the circulation and lessen the visions in some people with Lewy body dementia. While some of these people may have truly disturbing visions, in my practice I have rarely had to prescribe antipsychotic drugs, and in those who are also taking anti-Parkinson drugs, reducing that medication will often reduce or eliminate the visions.

It is important to emphasize that dementia is *not* a psychiatric illness. Broadly applying labels that relate to psychiatric illness produces a mindset that leads us to use drugs that have little benefit and high risk.

In his book *Hallucinations*, Sacks (2012) describes many of the "hallucinations" of dementia as "embedded in a complex matrix of sensory deceptions, confusion, disorientation, and delusions" (p.88). It is heartening to see a published quote from a well-respected neurologist that approaches my contention that we are overapplying the concept of psychosis in dementia. (In addition to describing an array of unusual and bizarre types of hallucinations in his book, Sacks also devotes a great deal of text to experiences that many of us without significant disease may encounter, and his examples challenge the idea that every strange perceptual experience requires medical intervention.)

"It's Me!"

As you can see, once we delve into the domain of meaning, the possibilities are as numerous as the people who express them. The preceding scenarios are only a sample of the various ways in which meaning can be expressed. Hopefully the examples discussed here will help the reader to see with new eyes and listen with new ears when partnering in care.

Before we move on to the topic of growth, I would like to share one more challenge. One common remark that is intended to reassure frustrated care partners is, "It's not him; it's the dementia speaking." I have never been a fan of this comment. I understand that it is intended to soothe the feelings of people who may be angry or hurt by what the person has said or done. The problem is that such a comment medicalizes the issue, once again blaming a damaged brain; as a result, we will look to chemical manipulation, rather than eroded well-being.

The truth is, it *is* the person speaking. We may not like the way he has expressed himself, but this is the best way he can tell us he has needs that are not being met. In "To Whom I May Concern" (Bowly, 2013), participant Steve echoes this view:

> I hear professionals saying stuff like, "It's the disease speaking." I want to yell, "No, it's not the disease speaking—it's me! Steve—father, husband, son, friend—Steve!"

As Naomi Feil (2002) reminds us:

> Painful feelings that are expressed, acknowledged, and validated by a trusted listener will diminish. Painful feelings that are ignored or suppressed will gain strength and can become "toxic." (p. 30)

CHAPTER 8

Growth

A ship in port is safe, but that's not what ships are built for.
—Grace Murray Hooper

If we don't change, we don't grow. If we don't grow, we are not really living. Growth demands a temporary surrender of security.
—Gail Sheehy

Well-being changes as we move through life, which is why a child's version of it cannot be the same as an old person's.
—Deepak Chopra

WE NOW COME TO THE domain that is usually most difficult to visualize. For those who have learned to view dementia primarily in terms of deficits and decline, the concept of growth must seem almost impossible. But hopefully the preceding chapters have shown that the various domains of well-being can be enhanced even for people with severe cognitive disabilities. And if enhancing identity, connectedness, security, autonomy, and meaning provides fertile soil for growth, then hopefully the reader can now begin to see this possibility as well.

In this chapter, we will look at shortcomings in the ways in which we view and measure growth, as well as the effects of stigmas related to aging and dementia. And we will share stories that show such growth occurring, even to the last days of life. As with previous chapters, this approach will challenge some of the ways we see and care for people, because this is a domain that is rarely considered when such practices are implemented.

Growth Defined

Fox et al. (2005) define growth as encompassing the following qualities: development; enrichment; unfolding; expanding; evolving. Immediately, these words run in direct opposition to the societal paradigm for viewing dementia: decline; limitation; misfolding (of brain proteins); contracting; and devolving to a child-like state.

How could these two views be so diametrically opposed? If you subscribe to the hierarchy displayed in my well-being pyramid (Figure 3), it is quite apparent. Since each successive level is influenced by those below it, the negative effects of stigma and potentially harmful care practices will have a cumulative effect as we climb the pyramid, just as wind causes a building to sway more at the top than at lower levels.

Like each previous level of the pyramid, there is another close pairing between meaning and growth. When we connect to those things that are meaningful, they enable us to grow—in ability, in creativity, in expressivity, in relationships, in spirituality.

We have built such a strong and detailed foundation to our pyramid that these last two well-being chapters will be a bit shorter. Many of the concepts from earlier chapters reappear in the latter domains and do not need repeating. However, do not assume that the issues described here will be less challenging; in fact, some of the greatest challenges to our attitudes and practices come out of these last domains.

Let us examine some of the factors that contradict a vision for growth. Then we will use all we have learned to construct an alternate vision—one that still holds the possibility of attaining self-actualization and joy.

How Dementia Challenges Growth

Intrinsic and Extrinsic Challenges

Once again, we will examine the intrinsic and extrinsic aspects in tandem. The first and most obvious challenge with dementia can be seen at the microscopic level. Brain cells are damaged; furthermore, this damage appears to be permanent and progressive for most people. In addition, the most common symptoms, such as memory loss, language difficulties, and impaired reasoning skills, appear to refute the possibility that a person can learn new information and become better at something than he was before. If brain cells are lost forever, and more brain cells are lost in the successive months and years, how can one possibly grow?

We have come back to the idea of cultural hegemony—a view of dementia put forth to society that sees only the aspects that reinforce the view. Our biomedical paradigm centers on the treatment of disease, and there is little room for a concept such as growth in a view defined by deficits and decline. We even perpetuate this narrow view in the ways in which we evaluate dementia.

First, we have discussed the standard cognitive assessments that measure discrete tasks and often miss more complex, integrative, or value-driven types of thinking. We use these tasks to place people into stages, creating generalizations for each stage that are defined primarily by what skills are lost. It is difficult for an individual to rise above such "pigeonholing":

> Taylor (2011) was once interviewed for a radio show. At one point, the host asked him what his current stage of Alzheimer's was. Taylor responded that he did not tend to dwell on such characterizations, but that by the usual staging system employed by the Alzheimer's Association, he guessed he would be considered Stage 4.
> The interviewer then asked, "Stage 4a, b, or c?"

Second, we also measure "behavior" purely in terms of negative experiences and expressions. Previously (Power, 2010), I reported that every published study of antipsychotic use in dementia has measured only the levels of negative symptoms, attempting to lessen their frequency with medication. Never has such a study attempted to measure any positive outcome of these drugs. A decreased level of distress does not equate to well-being.

Third, our brain scans have a similar shortcoming in evaluating people. Shabahangi (2014) explains what is missing:

> A neurologically normal brain might be regarded as healthy on a cat-scan display but it will say nothing whatsoever about the person's moral and ethical compass, that is if this person is a kind person or a dangerous criminal. Since we are not looking for a concept such as kindness, we do not even have an idea to look for it.
> . . . the world is seen through the lens of the data it demands. Much like the person who has lost his keys in the dark, and tries to find them only in illuminated spaces, so have we created a world where we

have stopped looking for the immeasurable exactly because it is not measurable (p. 214).

Keep in mind that the concept of cultural hegemony does not say that measurements such as a brain scan or cognitive test have no value. Rather, it says that in such a system these are the *only* dimensions that are regarded as valuable. In fact, there are few scales available that attempt to measure such positive attributes. I was part of a project team that created an assessment tool for The Eden Alternative® (which I will describe in Chapter 10), but the larger question is, why do so many people feel that we need to thoroughly measure such qualities *before* they will be considered important to pursue? What about the ethical imperative to provide humanistic care?

Imagine the following three scenarios: (1) you find a wallet on the sidewalk that contains a large amount of cash, credit cards, and a driver's license; (2) you are walking down the street, cell phone in hand, and you see a man lying on the grass clutching his chest and pleading for you to "get help"; (3) you are walking through a department store and see a crying child who tells you he has become separated from his mother. Would you know what to do in each scenario? Do you need to wait for an evidence-based study to tell you what to do?

What is the danger of embracing only a narrow, deficit-based view? Again, it is the self-fulfilling prophecy. If we do not expect that people can learn and grow, we will not create a care environment that enables them to do so, and their subsequent failure will reinforce our view that they are simply fading away.

The Problem with Retrogenesis

One view regarding people living with dementia is that they not only cannot grow, but they even undergo a kind of reverse growth, slowly losing their cognitive and functional abilities in the opposite order in which they were developed. Because many of the lost capabilities mirror levels of function that develop in childhood, this concept of "retrogenesis" sees people becoming child-like again, and often measures their "cognitive age" in this manner. In fact, many practitioners develop activities that are based on such a cognitive age. It is not uncommon to hear someone say, "He now has the brain of a 3-year-old, and so we have to relate to him in this manner."

I have a problem with this view. A person may have challenges with speaking, walking, or continence that resemble what we might see in a small child, but there are very important differences. First of all, each person follows a journey that is highly individualized. People rarely follow a straight path, or fit neatly into simple categories. Such a view obscures the individual.

But more important is the fact that an older person living with dementia has lived 60, 70, or 80 years or more. He has been to school, held a job, fallen in love, been sexually intimate, suffered loss and trauma, worked at an occupation, raised children. Regardless of what capabilities are lost, such a person will never view the world around him the same way a small child would.

An example is the experience of being bathed by a care partner, perhaps of the opposite sex. How would a typical 3-year-old experience this activity compared to an adult who has known body maturation, sexual intimacy, and perhaps even sexual assault? Even though memories and functional capacities may be lost, this does not mean that such a person would have the same response as the child.

Viewing an older person as we would a child simply because many of his abilities are at a similar level is another example of how we use narrow measurements to create sweeping generalizations about a person, often positioning him as being less capable than he truly is. And when we treat that person like a child, we often meet with resistance, as Davis describes when he critiqued some senior center activities in Chapter 7.

All of this brings us to the difficult subject of dolls, or even "doll therapy." This has been a concept I have struggled with for some time. Many women living with dementia have been given dolls to keep or carry with them. Indeed, I have seen many who appear affectionate, protective, and even happy when holding them. From the standpoint of my well-being approach, that might indicate that I should be accepting of the practice. But it has never felt quite right to me. The image of a grown woman holding a doll has often looked undignified to me; is that just my own judgment, or is there a deeper problem, even for the woman who appears contented?

I recently consulted Susan Frazier, COO of The Green House® Project, about this topic (knowing that she does not approve of the use of dolls), to hear her insights. She gave a very compelling reason why we should indeed be concerned about this. Frazier allows that dolls can have a role in settling a person's agitation, and even addressing an underlying need to nurture. And at times the person may not be fully aware of the difference between the doll and a live child. However,

Frazier believes that the fact that *we* know that there is a difference is important, because it can cause us to devalue the confused or child-like person. Our society's tendency to place more value on intellect and beauty feeds into a stigmatized view of such a person, which can affect our sense of her worth and, in turn, can subconsciously affect the many ways in which we interact with and care for her.

In other words, dignified, respectful care is more a function of how we see the person than how she sees herself, so the mere fact that she is not feeling undignified by the interaction may not be sufficient. This view directly supports the discussion of growth, as we are asserting that humans do not simply devolve on a downward spiral, but continue to have opportunities to develop. That may be harder to see when we position adults as children, and we may deny them those opportunities to continue to develop as adults.

There are also two other points to consider. The first is that the use of dolls to fulfill a need to nurture is somewhat similar to my point about having roommates to provide security; in this case, the Band-Aid is that we are providing a remedy for an environment that falls short of creating true nurturing. If we could create real caregiving opportunities for people with dementia (gardening, pets, interactions with children and babies, etc.) then the need for a doll would likely vanish.

> St. John's administrator Rebecca Priest caused a bit of a stir a few years ago when she brought her newborn daughter to work to visit a group of people living with advanced dementia. There was some concern expressed about the fact that she passed her baby to several of them to hold and cuddle. Rebecca reminded her colleagues that the ability to hold and nurture a small child is one of the most durable skills, even in people living with dementia, and they proved her right with their tender loving care.

There is a woman who moved from St. John's nursing home to one of their community Green House® homes who carried a doll regularly. She no longer does so, even though her overall condition has not changed appreciably. This supports the notion that her needs are being met in other ways that do not result in her needing an artificial form of nurturing.

The second point (which I will revisit in Chapter 9) is that joy is a bit different from the other domains, as it can be more transient and superficial at times. The mere sight of joy alone does not guarantee well-being. Therefore, a person holding a doll may be happy in the moment, but if other aspects of well-being (such as growth) are not being supported, then the approach is probably inadequate.

This is a very controversial topic, but this discussion represents the way in which I have challenged myself as I have explored the framework of well-being, and I invite others to do the same. And I will not even start in on the topic of robotic baby seals, which have been marketed as a therapeutic device to help comfort people with dementia.

Segregated Living and Growth

As noted previously, many of the stigmas already listed exist in all living environments. But the philosophy behind segregation can lead one to expect less, since the "disease" is the defining factor of the living area. If we concentrate on how a person with dementia might upset his cognitively able neighbors, instead of how he might learn and grow from interactions with them, we will never see the value of diverse engagement.

Such value also includes the enhanced meaning and growth experienced by the more cognitively able elders as they assist those who need more guidance. Greenwood (personal communication, October 27, 2013), for example, quotes a woman who shared her experience of helping another woman with dementia become acclimated after moving into an integrated area of the home:

> I said to her, "Let's go and have a talk," and I did that most days; and she said to me, "I dreaded coming in here, but since we've got together and talked, it's made all the difference." Now I like to talk; it's one of the few things I can do.

Furthermore, even though we may be very caring and compassionate, if we do so from an attitude of lowered expectations, we can create excess disability. This, in turn, increases our care burden and makes it even harder to create the kind of flexibility that enables autonomy, meaning, and growth.

One of the most powerful arguments against segregated living areas that I have heard speaks directly to the domain of growth and the self-fulfilling prophecy:

> I was facilitating a seminar and was asked my opinion about "memory care units." Knowing that my opinion was still very

much in the minority, I proceeded very cautiously, stating that I was not in favor of segregated living, and gave a few of my reasons. During the break that followed, my colleague, Wendy Vaughn, told me a story that greatly strengthened my resolve.

Wendy used to work at Rolling Fields, an excellent Eden Alternative–affiliated nursing home near Erie, Pennsylvania. Several years ago, the home had a neighborhood designated for people with "end-stage" dementia. The approximately three dozen people living in this area were all uncommunicative, nonambulatory, incontinent, and needed complete assistance with meals and other activities of daily living. They received palliative care, and people from other areas whose dementia progressed to an advanced stage were moved to this unit.

The care was very loving and attentive, but when the home started their Eden affiliation, they discussed the importance of continuous relationships and questioned their practice of moving people at a time when they were most vulnerable. A decision was made to stop moving people to this area. Furthermore, the segregated living arrangement was disbanded, and those who were living there were dispersed back throughout the other diverse areas of the home.

Can you guess what happened to the people from that unit after being moved? They became more alert, verbal, interactive, and participatory. The staff realized that, despite their kind care, they had expected "end-stage disease," and their system of care had deepened people's dependence and decline. No one would have expected the people from that unit to ever reverse any of their disability.

I will close out my argument for integration with two last points. One is that the percentage of people living with dementia in skilled or assisted living settings continues to increase—up to 70% or more in many countries. The idea of continuing to separate people in these settings is becoming more and more untenable.

For the last point, I will return to the "civil rights" argument I made in *Dementia Beyond Drugs*. For me, the argument against segregation always begins and ends here. There is no other population (outside of prisons) who are told they cannot live around the rest of us. I often engage participants in the following exercise:

In order to minimize the potential of offending anyone, I ask each person to silently choose a personal characteristic of his or her own, be it race, ethnicity, religion, or some other defining trait. As I recite the following statements, I ask each person to imagine I am referring to people who share the trait they have chosen:

"Others do not like having them in the same living area. They frighten the other residents, and their families complain. We find it's better to move them so that they can live separately. They need different activities, a different living environment, and a different approach to care. They won't bother each other as much as they bother other people. They will be much happier if they are around people of their own kind."

In this context, the preceding comments sound quite offensive, do they not? And yet, are they any different when referring to people living with dementia—people who are each as unique as the various members of any race or religious group?

Community-Based Living and Growth

Despite the advantages of living in the community (familiarity, diverse surroundings, tie-in to personal history, etc.), the stigmas regarding growth can also be stifling. O'Connor (Bartlett & O'Connor, 2010) regularly visited a woman living in her own home. The woman had a fair amount of forgetfulness, but was compensating for it and appeared to be doing quite well in this situation. O'Connor was later surprised to receive a copy of a formal neuropsychological assessment that highlighted the woman's illness and painted her as being largely incapable:

> I had been focusing on what Mrs. Wright could do—her strengths—the testing had revealed what she couldn't do—her deficits. . . . it was revealing to note that despite her appalling test scores, Mrs. Wright continued to live with relative safety in the community for an additional two years. (pp. 66–67)

The narratives I have shared of people who have lived with dementia show their struggles with these attitudes. In each case, the person reaches a greater understanding of his intrinsic value, one that his care partners may not have realized:

> In Alzheimer's you come back to being very childlike, like an infant in your ability to function. But value lies not in what you can do, but in your being. People are valuable for what they are in the present, not just for their pasts or for their future potential.

> We need to see the person with disease as being a complete person in the moment, not as being a partial person. That was the fallacy in Hitler's Nazism—seeing value only in the superman and disposing of all the others. It ended up destroying the culture. (Simpson, & Simpson, 1999, p. 122)

DeBaggio (2002) says it this way:

> Instead of becoming emotional about me and this brain disease, if my friends thought about it, Alzheimer's could be a liberating event, freeing me to float through life and stand it on its head. Come fly with me. (p. 48)

Through these narratives, we also see the close resonance between meaning and growth. People living with dementia are searching for the ongoing meaning in their lives, and in doing so are able to grow. Such a process can occur right to the end of one's life.

> Melanie Adair (SACFER, 2012) shares the story of Kathryn, who was 103 years old and lived with dementia in an assisted living home. She developed a close relationship with Janelle, her aide. Janelle would often help with Kathryn's insomnia by giving her hot cocoa or a back massage. Kathryn gave Janelle advice about her son's struggles in school, and they often prayed together.
>
> A few weeks before her death, Kathryn shared with Janelle that she had been raised in a manner that led her to dislike people of color, but that their relationship had changed that.
>
> Kathryn said, "I have been prejudiced my whole life about black people and now I know how wrong I was. I have prayed and asked God to forgive me. As soon as I did, I felt lighter than I have in years. My spirit soared in ways I didn't know were possible. My relationship with Janelle has truly changed my life." (p. 14)

Once again, the power of growth and development persists throughout one's life, despite significant cognitive disability. This is too often lost on those who know the person best. In a sad epilogue, after Kathryn's death, her family's eulogies spoke only about the Kathryn they had known years before, because they saw her as fading away and did not see the value in her last years.

Professionals working in community settings also fall prey to the same stigmas as their colleagues in long-term care. Shanks (1999) tells the story of a 96-year-old woman with Alzheimer's (Bessie) who lived with her daughter, Helen:

> Three years ago, Bessie was dismissed from the day-care center that she had attended for several years on the grounds that she was too fragile to continue. Yet although Bessie is very slow now, she is still able to walk, and since she was dismissed from the center, Helen has taken her on two plane trips to family reunions in California. . . . She did not feel that her mother's [Alzheimer's], even in the advanced stage, was a reason not to carry out her plans . . . and said that Bessie could now walk as far as two blocks. (p. 123)

Because of her daughter's belief in her ability to continue to engage and grow, Bessie had continued to experience life to her fullest extent, and her abilities improved as a result. These are examples of real growth, in even the most frail among us.

Enhancing Growth

I will outline several ways in which we can enhance growth via the three pathways of personal, operational, and physical transformation. As with the previous chapters, this list is not meant to be exhaustive, but it should give readers many avenues through which to explore the realms of possibility for the people they support.

Personal Transformation

Opening our eyes to the potential for growth begins by rejecting the view of dementia as one of pure decline. It should be fairly clear from our own lives that this is possible: as we pass through adulthood and our abilities and preferences evolve, we see ourselves losing some skills through aging, while growing and deepening our wisdom in other areas. The presence of physical or cognitive illness may heighten the challenge of growth, but it is far from impossible if those around us recognize and support the process.

Let us begin by looking at the positive aspects of living with cognitive illness. Are there any? Shabahangi (Voris, Shabahangi, & Fox, 2009) elaborates:

> Sometimes I ask a student, "Can you think of a part of your mind that would benefit (from living with cognitive loss)?" Almost always, students can find that part. For example, they would answer that they would like their inner critic to be less vocal, would love their inner taskmaster, the one who doesn't want you to sleep late, the one with the never ending "to do" lists, to be more quiet. (pp. 50–51)

In fact, I believe there are several areas in which people living with dementia are more skilled than the rest of us. One that we have already discussed is their sensitivity to nonverbal language—the ability to see what lies behind our words. Another is the ability to be in the moment. Many of us spend a lot of time and money studying mindfulness, yoga, meditation, or tai chi; yet a person living with dementia often has the ability to let go of intrusive thoughts and just be in the present moment, noticing little things that often escape our attention.

As I stated in the last chapter, I believe people living with dementia are often more motivated to look for meaning in their lives, and they teach us that we should begin this search before we are faced with serious illness. As a result, such people are also able to drop pretense and set priorities around what is truly important to them, regardless of the expectations of others.

> We suggest that some parts of our identity might even benefit from forgetting. Forgetting may allow for other, deeper parts of our identity to come to the foreground, parts our remembering keeps forgetting. The stories behind identity, behind remembering and forgetting, are not fixed but fluid; they depend much on our vantage point, our priorities, and our lives. (Shabahangi & Szymkiewicz, 2008, pp. 14–15)

Shanks (1999) relates a visit to a pair of elder sisters who imparted great wisdom to her for her years of caring for her husband:

> Sharon, one of the "sisters," told me, "As human beings, we have evolved physically, but we are still in prehistoric times when it comes to our mental development."
> . . . I do not believe the books have been written yet on what is possible for the physically healthy [Alzheimer's] patient—one who is not given tranquilizing drugs and who is accepted and treated like a human being in the community of family and friends. (p. 32)

The authors I have referenced who have lived with dementia have made several observations that show the growth they have experienced despite their disability. DeBaggio (2003) addresses his sensitivity to "invisible" aspects of the world around him:

> Alzheimer's has given me something wonderful. I hear and see things nobody else experiences. They are my truly unique experiences because they occur totally inside my mind and I am unable to define them or describe them. (p. 152)

And, in a visit to a favorite old fly-fishing spot, he explains how the skills he learned there prepared him for the challenges he would experience later in life:

> In a lonely place like Mossy Creek you confront failure and see fine things come from it, especially the desire to push ahead, no matter the barriers . . .
>
> It was at Mossy Creek many years ago on a frigid overcast winter day I devoted myself to emptiness and discovered its charm and necessity . . .
>
> It was here understanding, as singular and robust as a dust mote, began to take place inside me.
>
> It was here I imagined the stalactites that inhabited the deep caves nurturing the cold waters flowing steadily in silence.
>
> It was here I learned how to peel back layers of memory left in times unprepared for tomorrow. (pp. 171–172)

In the remarkable poem "Lost and Found" (published in Digh, 2008), David Hollies, who began to lose memory at age 50, concludes with a startling realization:

> It was then that I realized
> Being lost only has meaning
> When contrasted with
> Knowing where you are
> A presumption that slipped out of my life
> As quietly as smoke up a chimney
> For now I live in a less anchored place
> Where being lost is irrelevant
> For now, only when there is a need
> Do I discover where I am
> No alarm, no fear
> Just an unconscious check-in
> Like glancing in the rear-view mirror. (p. 2)

This reflects the way in which people with dementia re-prioritize life to enable well-being. Robert Simpson (Simpson & Simpson, 1999) puts it this way:

> You know how it is when you push and push yourself to do something and you just can't do it anymore, so finally you give up? It's easier! It frees you up to do what you can do without beating yourself. Life is easier for me now than it was before I knew I had Alzheimer's. (p. 128)

In his 2003 memoir, Rose shares his own process of inner growth, rejecting a "declinist" view expressed by his friend Stella, and helping his son Jeff to understand his perspective:

> Stella says that I have cut myself off from most people. To her I have reduced my basic needs to the point of just eating, sleeping, writing and listening to music. I suppose that is the way she sees it. To me, an extraordinary calm has descended over me.
>
> . . . I was telling my son, Jeff, just the other day that there is so much more to life than just the quest for knowledge and wealth. Learning about kindness, courage and love are paramount. That is something that has to come from inside a person. You can't learn these things from books. (p. 46)

Many of the truths expressed in these quotes may seem self-evident, but our lack of mindfulness as we go about our days leads us to lose track of these principles in the ways in which we interact with others. Many people who live with dementia are able to focus much more intently on these aspects of life; in this way, they can acquire a Zen-like quality, cultivating an inner sense of truth and peace. And this, in turn, leads to insights that encompass people with more advanced disability, beyond the ego to something much deeper:

> Suppose my mind became so still that even the sense *I* was gone. . . . There would be no grasping after I and mine, just a brilliant clarity. There would be total freedom in this clear, empty, unimpeded cognition. (Voris et al., 2009, pp. 69–70, emphasis added)

Thoughts such as these reflect the third part of the dementia journey described by Bryden: moving into spirit. While highly individualized and tied to faith traditions, the notion of spirit (or soul) has a place in most people's belief systems. While Voris's statement brings to mind a Zen philosophy, the story of Kathryn displayed personal growth rooted in her Christian faith. In both cases, the person's spirituality is an important pathway to growth.

Here is how Simpson (Simpson & Simpson, 1999), a Christian pastor, counters the retrogenesis view of dementia that was presented to him:

> As I was thinking about this apparent regression, and feeling sad about it, I thought about becoming a child. I recalled Jesus' words, "Unless you become as a little child, you can never enter the King-

dom of Heaven." I found this reassuring. Even if I am losing much of myself, I am not outside of God's love. I may be even closer than before. (p. 76)

Wong (2009) tells of his mother's indomitable spirit, even evident after she became uncommunicative:

> Just three days ago Ma seemed to have discarded the spirituality so characteristic of her. Now I found out that silence and stillness did not mean absent spirituality. A new lesson from my dying mother. (p. 170)

Care Partner Growth

Another often-overlooked aspect of growth is the experiences of care partners of those who live with dementia. Many narratives express the challenges and the upheavals of life when a loved one develops a cognitive disability. But such challenges are also opportunities for growth, and with the sadness and loss comes a wisdom and even an appreciation for having gone through the experience. Shouse (2006) wrote a memoir of caring for her mother, a story heavy with sadness and loss. And yet, in her mother's final days, she reflects:

> By allowing myself to contemplate and discuss my mother's impending death, I have enriched my life and the life that she has left. (p. 161)

> I am still receiving richness from our relationship, beyond what I thought was possible. I would never have guessed that I could sit on the edge of a hospital bed with a non-communicative woman and still feel the warmth of connection. (p. 167)

In some cases, even people who have advanced cognitive disability explicitly teach lessons to their care partners. Wong (2009) tells the story of coming to his mother's apartment and finding that her aide, Karma, had left her unattended. He became very upset and confronted the woman angrily when she returned. This greatly upset his mother, who expressed her unhappiness with his behavior, and made him apologize to Karma:

> "Any problem, slowly explain for her to understand," she said. "Yes she is wrong in going out for so long. But you are wrong for shouting, for being so aggressive. . . . "

It was the cusp of late-stage Alzheimer's. Yet Ma displayed moral outrage, stopped my unbridled anger, and pressed me into contrition. Ma had always urged me to respect people, whatever their status and station. . . . The neural connectors had frayed, but her moral fibres were intact. (pp. 141–142)

Shanks (1999) shares the lessons she learned about her own barriers to understanding, as well as how she became enlightened by the experience of caring for her husband, Hughes:

I can now say that Hughes is often the least of my difficulties, primarily because my resistance to caring for him is so much lessened. Often it is not so much the tasks themselves as our resistance to them that causes us stress and wears us down. (p. 65)

Careproviding presents us with the challenge of a lifetime, and the hardest task many of us will ever face. But the extraordinary circumstances in which it places us are also opportunities to open up to new frontiers in human development and understanding. (p. 82)

Hughes' illness forced me to discover a whole new part of myself I never knew existed. It is as if he had to become incapacitated in order for me to grow in unknown and unexplored areas of self-realization. (p. 113)

Many who tell such stories acknowledge the hardships, but state that they would never trade the experiences they had for a life of greater ease. The knowledge of the finitude of life helps both the person living with the disorder and his care partner to understand how to appreciate and celebrate each moment.

Shabahangi (2014) shares how a woman in her late thirties who had cared for her father for 8 years addressed a workshop audience:

She remarked that in the first 6 years she envied her peers who were pursuing careers, family, travel, and other more mainstream pleasures. Only in her last 2 years of care-taking did she recognize, so she said, that she was the lucky one, that she had been privileged with the profound experience that came with the task of having to care so deeply for a loved one. . . . She spoke glowingly about all her dad was teaching her everyday as she had to bathe, dress, groom, and feed him. She said that she was learning about love, learning about being in the moment with him and herself, about going slow, about being kind and caring, about being attentive to the little things. After the room had fallen very quiet, she said that for her caring for someone else felt like the most precious gift she could have been given in life. (pp. 213–214)

"Brain Fitness"

I would like to offer one more opinion on the subject of personal growth and cognitive disorders. I am often asked what I think of "cognitive enhancing" exercises and the explosion of resources around this concept.

I think there is ample evidence that keeping one's brain active is good for cognitive health. It also appears that challenging our minds to think in novel ways can also expand our capabilities. However, as I stated earlier, my personal feeling is that we should engage in activities that are meaningful and relevant for us. If you do not enjoy Sudoku puzzles, do not do them. Better to engage a friend in conversation about something that is important to you, to buy that book you always wanted to read, to volunteer at your local school, or to take those piano lessons you regret not having taken in childhood, than to spend your days aimlessly looking at flash cards and word games. I consider meaning and growth to be essential to optimizing our health and well-being.

George & Whitehouse (2011) see the brain fitness craze as emblematic of a reductionistic view of brain health that has occurred as an outgrowth of our biomedical model. It presumes that science and technology will create well-being and that the individual holds the power to create his own future brain health. And it also feeds on our deep fear of losing our memories.

The authors point out that it is normal for a skill to improve with repetition. The larger question is whether these activities, often performed in isolation, will impact one's future well-being in meaningful ways. With regard to this question, the research has been less than overwhelming. The authors point to The Intergenerational School in Cleveland, Ohio (described later in this chapter), as an example of a more meaningful approach to cognitive enhancement that engages the generations in shared learning activities.

For my money, any intellectual exercise that harnesses the domains of well-being is much more likely to create a durable form of brain health. In addition, it creates meaning for the person doing it, strengthening the value of the activity for the lives of the person and those with whom he engages. And the truth is, many people will eventually develop forgetfulness in advanced age, even if they keep their brains active; it is far better that they enter that phase of life knowing how to live meaningfully. So put away the flash cards, and get involved with your neighbors or your community.

Operational Transformation

Once we have reaffirmed the possibility of growth for people living with dementia and their care partners, our systems of support and care must enable such growth potential to be optimized. And even though we are talking about systems and operations, remember that these concepts apply to all living settings, including one's own home.

Operations that support growth are those in which the person has the opportunity to *be* useful, not just to *feel* useful. Growth also occurs in the sharing of wisdom with others, and even in the stillness of being.

We discussed examples of activities that create meaning in Chapter 7. Each of these is a path to growth as well. This growth is more than an internal process of self-actualization; like Bessie, who was "expelled" from the day center, we can even see improvements in physical and cognitive abilities.

A key is to use an approach to activities that builds on existing strengths, rather than one that is purely defined by, or formulated to improve, deficits. One strength retained by many people is the ability to read, even when speaking becomes impaired. Camp (2102) gives several examples of how the use of signs and printed material can be successfully used for cueing, engagement, or sharing other important information.

> The ability to read is usually retained even when a person has dementia. Reading might be elicited through printed words even if the person with dementia is usually nonverbal. It is such a well-practiced habit that we don't even think about it while we do it, and this habit may still be available in advanced stages of dementia. Never assume that persons cannot read just because they have dementia. (pp. 35–36)

Another strength is the ability to engage in narrative. We have discussed the importance of narrative in helping people express their feelings, and its use as a foundation for Anne Basting's TimeSlips™ approach. Camp (2012) gives an example of how the use of narrative helped a disengaged woman to reconnect. Her daughter was frustrated because her visits to the nursing home elicited little meaningful conversation from her mother. Working with the activity professional, they developed a different approach that leaned on narrative:

> On her next visit, the daughter said, "Mom, tell me a story about when you were four years old." The older woman thought a bit, and with some prompting began to tell a story. The daughter wrote it down. Then, the daughter said, "Mom, tell me a story about something I did when I was four years old." The older woman thought a bit, and then related a relevant story. Again, the daughter wrote it down. (p. 38)

Using an appropriate font size and style, the daughter printed the stories on sheets of paper, which she passed to her 4-year-old granddaughter to illustrate with crayon drawings. She then returned to the nursing home with her granddaughter and the stories:

> The older woman with dementia read the stories out loud to her great-granddaughter. Children love to hear family stories, especially about little children their own age. When finished, the little girl asked her to read the stories again.
>
> This created a different kind of visit for the grown daughter and her mother. It allowed the older woman to become the keeper of family history and the teller of stories. It allowed her grown daughter to have more enjoyable visits and a close relationship with her mother. It allowed the great-granddaughter to have pleasant visits as well, and to have a relationship with the older woman. The nursing home was neither scary nor boring to the child in this context. (p. 39)

In this case, the woman had difficulty with verbal expression in normal conversation, but her narrative and reading skills were very much preserved. By tapping into these skills, and adding meaning and connectedness through her great-granddaughter's artwork and participation as an audience, an important role was re-established for the woman.

By tying into past history and bringing important aspects of identity forward, people who have become disengaged can re-emerge and show their potential for growth. During one of my seminars, an educator who supports several homes in the midwestern United States shared the following story of a consultation she had with the staff of one nursing home:

> The staff were frustrated with a gentleman who had moved in not long before. His overall demeanor was seen to be nasty and uncooperative; he declined all programmed activities, ate meals alone in his room, and often resisted attempts to help him with care.
>
> The educator began by visiting with the gentleman for about 15 minutes, to get to know him a bit. She emerged from the

room and asked the staff members what they knew about the man. The staff responded that they knew very little about him and that he was "just nasty." She said, "Did you know that he is a retired engineer and he was involved with designing the It's a Small World ride at Disneyland?"

The staff members were dumbfounded to hear of this history; stuck in the usual paradigm of caring for the person who challenges, they failed to appreciate that he could have a history rich with accomplishments. The educator suggested that they engage him in conversation on this topic. When they did so, he began to visibly brighten, his demeanor became more pleasant and animated, and he told stories of his past work.

The man's story was shared with other staff, and the maintenance workers began to invite him to join them when working on projects around the home. He would sit and observe their work and add his thoughts on their projects. He was asked to share his story with other elders as well, and he gradually began to engage with the life of the home. Eventually, he became much more involved in activities, joined the communal meals, and had a remarkable change in his overall mood and disposition.

This story reminds us of the interplay between the various domains of well-being. The path to growth for this gentleman was particularly tied to identity, connectedness, and meaning. One can also predict that the staff's limited view of him had contributed to an erosion of security and autonomy in daily life as well. More important, this story shows the powerful effect the care partners' attitude and approach can have in eroding or enabling a person's well-being.

Another simple but powerful way to enable meaning and growth is to involve people in discussions and solicit their input. This goes beyond simply being invited to join a care plan meeting (although all too often people are even excluded from these); it also involves joining meetings to discuss and plan daily life in the home, and participating on planning committees for renovations, celebrations, and other initiatives.

In Chapter 7, I shared the story of a woman at SentryCare in Mississippi who during a group interview conveyed her very frank opinions of a prospective employee. Another interview story from SentryCare involves a woman who spent most of her days insulting everyone with whom she came into contact. Her language was quite colorful; the staff said that she had taught them a few new words! Rather than expressing shock or anger, the staff continued to engage her and usually looked humorously at her liberal use of "sailor's language."

The staff decided to invite her to join one of their group interviews. (In retrospect, I am not sure if they had high expectations of her, or if they thought her language might be a good way to test the composure of the interviewee.) In any event, the interview proceeded smoothly; the woman made a couple of appropriate comments, but otherwise sat quietly and did not use any foul language.

Surprised, one of the staff members addressed her after the interview and observed that she had not cursed once during the meeting. The woman looked at her as if she were a little dense and matter-of-factly replied, "I know how to behave during an interview!"

While this story is humorous on the surface, there is another point that should not be missed. What has been viewed as a "dementia-related behavior" was entirely suppressed when she was given a meaningful role. This should tell us a great deal about the potential for people to maintain or grow skills when presented with diverse engagement, including sharing meaningful activity with cognitively normal people.

In Chapters 5 and 6, we discussed the interplay between security and autonomy, the problem of surplus safety, and the need to negotiate risk. Another benefit of negotiating risk is the potential for growth. Growth does not occur without change, or without some degree of risk:

> I had the opportunity to visit Mercy Parklands Nursing Home in Auckland, New Zealand, to observe their *Spark of Life* club in action. Before the meeting, a few staff members joined me for lunch, including Catherine Heaney, an occupational therapist who works at the home. She was showing me around the home when a woman living with dementia walked past us using a rolling walker. We greeted her as she went past.
>
> Catherine mentioned that the woman had become chair-bound after coming to the home, as her cognitive disability progressed. Her routine was to propel herself around the hallways in a wheelchair, using her feet.
>
> One day, Catherine walked past her and saw her tentatively stand up from the chair. Fighting the urge to run over and sit her back down, Catherine instead walked up to the woman, greeted her warmly, and said, "You are standing up. Do you want to walk?"
>
> The woman nodded and the staff began to work with her. The result was that several months later she was now walking independently. If no one had taken the chance and had just sat her back down, assuming that the risk of falling was too great, she never would have had the opportunity to regain her lost skill.

Returning to community-based living, growth also has the potential to broaden our paradigm beyond the world of providing "care." Bartlett and O'Connor (2010) assert that our current view of personhood is concerned more with *maintaining* status than with *enabling* growth and development:

> We do not know yet how to accommodate the notion that, like any-one else, people with dementia may change—they may change their mind, they may want to experiment, they may legitimately lose inter-est in activities that once enthralled them. . . . [T]here has been a tendency to conceptualise personhood in a way that may inadver-tently collude with the biomedical model to effectively discount people with dementia by relegating change to the neuropathological changes associated with the dementia rather than normal lifecourse maturation. (pp. 22–23)

Later, they add that in a larger "social citizenship" context

> the idea of "growth" is an important one, as it recognises a person's inner hopes, desires and capacity to contribute to life. From this per-spective "growth" means to be able to develop different aspects of oneself in the context of having one aspect deteriorating. (p. 40)

Here, then, is another challenge to the notion that people deteriorate continuously in all aspects when living with degenerative illness. Dif-ferent aspects of personhood can be developing just as others are de-clining or being cast off. Once again, a glance at our own growth and maturation shows this to be true, but the stigma of dementia keeps us from seeing a similar process in those affected.

All of the avenues for increasing meaning that we discussed in the last chapter will also help people to grow in community life. Mike Howorth (Howorth, Keady, Riley, & Drummond, 2012), another ex-ample of a person living with dementia, has taken social citizenship to the next level:

> Mike Howorth of Salford, part of greater Manchester, England, was diagnosed with Alzheimer's in 2007 while in his late seventies. In 2010, he began work as a facilitator for Greater Manchester's Open Doors Network, which had been created to support the mental health needs of the region. Keenly aware of his experiences after his diagnosis, Howorth recognized the need to reach out to others in his situation and provide

education, support, and encouragement to find opportunities for meaningful engagement in their community.

Howorth helps to organize "friendship support group" meetings, a "post-diagnostic support group" meeting, and an "Open Doors dementia café," where any interested citizen can obtain more information about dementia. He explains that while the National Dementia Strategy has a platform of valuing people living with dementia, it "does not give enough emphasis on empowering people with dementia themselves to take charge of their own futures and form supportive services on their own terms, with their own objectives. In short, people with dementia still appear to be 'done to' rather than 'done with.'" (p. 40)

In contrast, Howorth asserts, the new narrative "challenges the old discourse with its emphasis on describing the person with dementia's deficits, losses and the 'burdens' that they pose to others around them, to a 'new discourse', one where emphasis is placed upon what the person with dementia can still do, and more importantly, can still become." (p. 41)

In Cleveland, Ohio, Peter and Cathy Whitehouse helped establish "the world's first intergenerational charter school" (Whitehouse & George, 2008, p. 143). The Intergenerational School is an environment in which children ages 6 to 12 attend school where they regularly interact with older adults—adult education students, volunteers, and also people living with dementia. The elders mentor the children in a number of activities, from reading to computer skills to gardening. Whitehouse, a neurologist who has done extensive research into treatments for Alzheimer's, believes that "volunteering can be more cognitively enhancing than any pill an older person can put in their body" (p. 146).

The Intergenerational School also creates a vehicle for elders to share their wisdom with younger members of the community. We will expand on this concept in Chapter 11, when we look to the future of global aging and discuss innovative responses to our changing demographics.

Physical Transformation

Many of the attributes of the physical environment needed to promote growth have been addressed as components of support for the first five domains of well-being. Some of these include an environment that supports the evolving self by not only connecting to one's past, but also facilitating active engagement in the present (e.g., scale and design that encourage one to strive for greater independence of movement; removal of trappings that reinforce the "sick role" and foster dependency; familiarity of surroundings; and aspects that offer opportunities for meaningful activity).

To the previous discussion, I would like to add two further points. The first is flexibility. If one is to be able to change, experiment, evolve, or reinvent oneself, the design of the physical environment must be sufficiently flexible to enable *possibility*. This means an environment that can adapt to changing needs and abilities, using more of a "universal design" concept. If the structure is inflexible, attempts to grow will meet resistance and be stifled.

This issue flows into a second, very important concept, which I first learned of while working with Dr. Emi Kiyota, an environmental gerontologist and founder and president of the nonprofit organization Ibasho. During a 2012 Bellagio residency supported by the Rockefeller Foundation, Kiyota and I worked in partnership to develop guiding principles for her organization's mission to create "socially integrated and sustainable communities that value their elders" (www.ibasho. org), as well as to develop her idea for a vehicle for community integration, the Ibasho Café.

The Ibasho Café serves as a conduit for meaning and growth and is designed to re-engage elders with their larger communities. The café is an informal gathering place for the local community, where the elders are not only welcome as patrons, but also manage the café, serving drinks and snacks to other visitors. The café has multigenerational conveniences, such as wireless Internet and a children's library, to attract a diverse group to the setting.

The Ibasho Café is *not* a "senior center," nor does it offer an array of structured activities. It is meant to be organic, culturally appropriate, and community driven. Each person can contribute in a way that supports his or her own well-being.

The café creates opportunities for meaning and growth, and can also be designed to address a larger community need. The first Ibasho Café opened in 2013 in Ofunato, Japan, as a vehicle for helping restore a community largely destroyed by the 2011 earthquake and tsunami. Other cafés may serve other needs, such as providing positive role models for youths at risk. But the key is to keep it as organic as possible, and to avoid having operations and planning driven by outside "experts."

One of the guiding principles that Kiyota brought to the discussion in developing her idea for the café is the concept of embracing imperfection gracefully, which is best encompassed by the Japanese term *wabi sabi*. True beauty lies in imperfection, just as the beauty of delicate rice paper arises from the various shapes, colors, and textures within. Imperfection can also represent that which is unfinished, or which shows the effects of the passage of time. (These qualities can also be applied to older adults, who may be imperfect, or may live with illness, yet are still "unfinished" and capable of growth.) While the concept of embracing imperfection gracefully may be unfamiliar, it is an important one for us to understand, because it explains another subtle but powerful way in which we erode meaning and growth, especially in elder living communities.

Because we see the person as needing care, and focus on providing for all of her needs, we design living spaces that provide as perfect an environment as possible—perfectly shaped, perfectly equipped, perfectly safe. In this way, we feel we have done all we can to create well-being; however, this can actually have the opposite effect.

The rush to create perfection in a building or community is a slippery slope to institutionalization, because it leads us to make assumptions and generalizations about what people will need and to create an environment that does not require its inhabitants to engage for the purpose of improvement. They then reside in a place in which all the planning has been done for them, and they have no useful role.

A better approach is to leave the design and construction *intentionally unfinished*; that is, to leave certain features open to discovery and adjustment as the elders and their care partners live and work in the space and learn how it can better meet their unique rhythms and desires. Décor and furniture arrangements may be left to the residents to decide, and outdoor areas, such as gardens and walkways, may be left unfinished so that the elders have a purposeful way in which to contribute to the ongoing life of the home. Not only does this create opportunities for meaning and growth, it truly places decisions about the design and operation of the home in the hands of those who will live and work there.

Kiyota reminds us that we all live in places that are "works in progress," gradually improving or updating our houses and apartments as our needs and desires change, and as our budget allows. This is normalcy; anything that strives for perfection becomes artificial and, therefore, meaningless.

McKnight & Block (2010) echo this philosophy in describing how the systems approach to community tries to create order and solve everyone's problems for them, thus disengaging people and creating solutions that end up not having individual value:

> Systems that are constructed for order cannot provide satisfaction in domains that require a unique and personal human solution. . . .
>
> What happens in system life is that we become the system that we inhabit. We become replicable. We are interchangeable parts. . . .
>
> In system life, we must betray what is unique and personal about us, that which is the sum and substance of what builds relationships. If consistency is the system's strength, then the cost to our humanity is a system's weakness. . . .
>
> As soon as you create a world that ensures sameness and predictability, you have created conditions where the real humanity of citizens and employees is marginalized. (pp. 31, 32, 35)

Lastly, two additional ways to promote growth within the physical design are (1) to ensure those who will live and work there are actively engaged in the planning of the building or renovation, and (2) to connect a physical environment that supports growth with operational features that do the same.

Kiyota has created a process called *pre-design* in which organizations meet to discuss their mission, vision, and values; clarify their goals for a new living space; and explore the ways in which the space will be used in daily life *before* planning the walls and rooms. The building, Kiyota explains, is like a glove, and the operations and activities of daily life are the hand that moves the glove. The glove must be designed to fit the hand, or it will stifle normal life within the home, just as ski mittens would hamper the ability of surgeons to practice their craft.

Before we move on to the domain of joy, one last thought: The examples of growth listed in this chapter not only resonate with meaning, they also feed back into the earlier domains, creating a cycle of growth and self-actualization. Growth, in fact, is an important factor in the very first domain of identity, as it directly supports and maintains the evolving self.

The narratives I have shared show that as those who live with cognitive disorders work to discover meaning and growth, they reaffirm their personhood and create a level of comfort in the lives they are living. Reminiscent of Gloria Steinem's famous remark about her age, Robert Simpson (Simpson & Simpson, 1999) comments, "People say to me, 'You don't look like you have Alzheimer's!' I tell them, '*This* is what Alzheimer's looks like!'" (p. 158).

CHAPTER 9

Joy

Ecstasy is
The lilting cadence of a song
Lingering after the music ends.
The sigh of utter bliss. Content.
When love too over long
Held back, is finally spent.

—Elbirda Coveny

I MET ELBIRDA EARLY IN my nursing home career. She was born in the coal mining hills of West Virginia at the beginning of the 20th century. Her parents always loved the name Alberta, but being unschooled, they misspelled it when they named their newborn daughter.

Elbirda lived at the nursing home primarily because of physical frailty, with a small degree of forgetfulness. I stopped by for a routine visit one day and noticed the pen and notebook on her bedside table. When I asked about it, she told me that she liked to write poetry.

Based on the spelling of her name and her upbringing, I had a certain view of Elbirda, and I am sure my reply was friendly but patronizing. I expected something at a third-grade level of writing; but I had the good sense to ask if I could see a sample. She showed me the poem above—simple, yet profound; plain, yet elegant; short, yet complete. I was stunned, and properly chastened for rushing to judgment.

Joy Defined

Fox et al. (2005) define joy as "happiness; pleasure; delight; contentment; enjoyment." While the other domains often lead sequentially to one another, it can be said that all lead to joy. Joy is perhaps the ultimate outcome, the one that is most able to transcend ability and disability.

Joy, as mentioned in the last chapter, is also more fleeting when well-being is not fully supported. A person mired in grief or clinical depression can smile or laugh from time to time, but such moments are short-lived and belie the underlying sadness that pervades her life. Therefore, although joy can exist in a small moment, we also need to be sure that those moments of joy we see are not merely a respite from an overarching sense of loss; rather, we must cultivate the other six domains of well-being so that joy can be sustained. In this way, the opposite happens: instead of joy being a brief departure from sadness, it can become a durable strength that actually helps people through the inevitable sadness and loss that we all must face at times.

Throughout the discussion of the first six well-being domains, many recurrent themes have emerged. The nature of joy is such that it can rise and fall on the tide of how these other domains are enhanced. For that reason, I will not spin this chapter out in the same degree of detail, but will use the concept of joy to wrap up our discussion of these seven domains. Then, in Chapter 10, I will demonstrate a way to use these to understand distress that is radically different from the approach most people follow.

How Dementia Challenges Joy

In this section, I will combine all living environments, because there are fewer experiences that are specific to one environment or another. Joy is, in many respects, a final common pathway; so even though the other well-being domains may be experienced in slightly different ways in different locales, the net outcome will often be the same.

The intrinsic challenges to joy lie in the various capabilities that are affected. Forgetfulness takes away the ability to call up joyful experiences of the past and connect them to the present. Difficulties with comprehension, expression, and executive function all inhibit the ability to experience or express joy to the fullest as well.

But a lack of enjoyment is not an intrinsic feature of most forms of dementia. Even people who have blunted emotional expressions may nevertheless experience joy. To truly erode joy, extrinsic factors must come into play.

The first extrinsic factor experienced by people living with dementia is the sense of grief and loss that accompanies the diagnosis. While the illness is real enough, the prevailing societal view of dementia enhances one's sorrow, due to the negative images and stigmas regarding life with dementia. Our fear of dementia is so great that it is hard to imagine anyone who would not be despondent after receiving the news that they were showing unmistakable symptoms of the condition.

Complicating this expected grief is the burden of stigma, well described in the previous chapters. The stigmas of dementia, combined with a narrow biomedical approach, erode joy by eroding each of the supporting domains. So a loss of recognition of the person and of meaningful relationships, a lost sense of security, removal of autonomy and choice, meaningless days, and lack of opportunities to grow all rob the person of opportunities for joy.

And yet many of those who live with dementia have found a path to joy by finding meaning and opportunities for growth. In doing so, they show us that it is possible to live positively with cognitive disabilities. As mentioned in Chapter 8, Simpson (Simpson & Simpson, 1999) observes that making do with less can have a freeing effect. Voris (Voris, Shabahangi, & Fox, 2009) reflects, "When I received the information from my doctor that I had dementia, I was about as low as a snake's neck. But then it's been one generous thing after another" (p. 99). Voris (Voris et al., 2009) also observes that some of the losses he experienced brought unexpected benefits, once he adjusted to his "new normal":

> So in many ways, my life is richer because I don't have a car.
> There are more people in my life. And not driving a car gives me a picture of a world that I didn't see when I was driving. Each day when I walk, I see and hear all the birds and animals that I didn't see and hear before. I don't think it's misleading to say I'm unquestionably happier and fuller with less. (p. 57)

Granted, joy is easier to attain when one has an inner predisposition to view the world from a positive standpoint. Many people living with Alzheimer's find joy in every day, while many others who are completely healthy seem to be miserable most of the time. Anne Simpson (Simpson & Simpson, 1999) explains it this way:

> A young doctor in our community was killed with her family in a tragic auto accident three years ago. The last entry written in her journal was, "Joy is a decision." It is Bob's decision. I pray that it can be mine as well. (p. 155)

And Shanks (1999) agrees:

> Joy, like patience and courage, faith and hope, is an inner strength that comes with us at birth . . . But like attitude, joy is a matter of our choice. It requires nothing of us except our acceptance. (p. 115)

People such as Ed Voris and Bob Simpson seem to rise above the challenges presented to them with amazing strength and resolve. But they, and many others, need our help to maintain the experience of joy. It is imperative that we work to remove the stigmas and create the conditions necessary to foster well-being.

It is very important that we do not make assumptions about the quality of life of a group of people, based simply on their cognitive or functional scores. Many studies (e.g., Sands et al., 2004) show that families and professional care partners consistently rate the quality of life of people with dementia lower than those people rate themselves. Studies also show that the self-rating of quality of life for people living with dementia is most correlated with their mood, whereas family members often project their own quality of life and care burden onto their assessments of loved ones, and the ratings made by professional staff are biased by their view of the person's degree of dependency (Hoe et al., 2006, Arons et al., 2013).

Enhancing Joy

Since joy often results from optimization of the other domains, let us review the basic approaches for each that will help create joy. I will then discuss a few other areas that can be particularly valuable to consider.

1. *Identity:* Knowing the person well and understanding what brings her pleasure helps us to personalize activities and interactions.

2. *Connectedness:* Cultivating close, meaningful relationships brings the joy of having trusted friends and confidantes. Being connected to one's past and to the intangible can also bring moments of joy.

3. *Security:* Familiarity and trust build a sense of security, which in turn enables a person to be free from fear and open to joy. Finding the right mix of spontaneity and routine enables the unexpected to create pleasant surprises and delights.

4. *Autonomy:* Having choice and control over a situation gives a person more ability to create engagement that fits his needs, abilities, and individual rhythms. Negotiating risk also enables access to joys that might be unattainable in a more restrictive environment.

5. *Meaning:* Being engaged in activities that speak to one's personal history and values is essential to daily enjoyment and fulfillment.

6. *Growth:* There is joy in accomplishment and self-actualization—in engaging with the world in all its variety and becoming more today than you were yesterday.

Here is the foundation, but there are some other ways in which we can also contribute to joy. Each of them can be adapted to a person's individual needs and abilities and requires relatively little time and effort.

Simple Pleasures

One way to bring about joy and create connections to earlier life is through the exploration of simple pleasures. These are exactly as they sound—simple activities or experiences that bring pleasure to the person. We all have them. They could be as varied as playing with a child, sitting with a cup of coffee and watching the sunrise, singing, or taking a bubble bath.

The key is that they are simple and can be engaged in without great time or expense. Also, they are very specific to the person; this is how meaning and joy are created. The little details are important, because they give it the special, personal touch. A cup of coffee, for example, needs to be the kind a person likes, prepared as she likes it, in the right cup or mug, at the time that she wants to drink it. (There are probably a number of coffee drinkers reading this who can attest to the importance of "doing it correctly.")

Of course, in the traditional nursing home, a simple pleasure is not always so simple. In the preceding example, a person may want the coffee at a time when the morning meal is not ready to be served. A special mug may have to be washed for the person's use, and the timing of arising may need to be shifted to accommodate the early hour. As you can see, an institutional home may need to shift a lot of operations just to accommodate this "simple" request.

As we discussed in the chapters on security and autonomy, if the task seems daunting, start with one person at a time, one simple pleasure at a time. The learning curve will be cumulative, and the effect of such a small change on the person can be dramatic, which will encourage the home to continue the process for others.

While they may be termed simple pleasures, their effect is anything but small. In the book, *Old Age in a New Age: The Promise of Transformative Nursing Homes* (Baker, 2007), culture change specialist Steve Shields of Action Pact, Inc., tells the story of Ida, a 100-year-old resident of Meadowlark Hills Nursing Home in Manhattan, Kansas. She was known for her unpleasant disposition and her frequent insulting comments directed toward those around her. Shields, who was Meadowlark's CEO at the time, decided to take her on as his "culture change project." He asked her to name anything she wanted to do for a day and he would try his best to grant it.

> He was prepared to fly to Paris with Ida, he claims, if that was her heart's desire. But Ida couldn't come up with anything she wanted. He told her he would give her more time to think about it. He returned the next day, but to his disappointment she said, "I'm too far gone." (p. 60)

Shields's colleague, LaVrene Norton, heard his tale of woe and informed him that a full day was too overwhelming to offer a woman who had had so little choice for years. She suggested he go back and ask Ida how she would spend just 5 minutes, any time of day:

> She didn't hesitate. She said she would watch the sunrise and drink a cup of her favorite tea in a Staffordshire china cup. That was the kind of china her mother had.
>
> He had to buy a set of eight, Steve said, but it was worth it. From then on, Ida woke at dawn, gazing out the large windows at the field surrounding Meadowlark and sipping Earl Grey tea in a Staffordshire china teacup. Such a simple daily ritual, but one that she had not been able to enjoy since moving to the nursing home. (p. 60)

Shields later observed that this simple pleasure was transformative for Ida. Her disposition changed completely, and she became a favorite of the staff members. This example shows the creation of joy, but also the ties to autonomy, connectedness, and meaning through the establishment of an important daily ritual. The tea was enjoyed in a cup that tied Ida to her mother and her upbringing, and was experienced at a time of day when she felt particularly reflective. Shields concluded his vignette by asking the readers, "How much have we been taking away from people, in our blindness" (p. 60)?

Laughter

Many people who live with dementia have a great capacity to laugh. Laughter can release pent-up emotions and defuse stressful situations. Laughter releases endorphins, and its effect on a group of people is contagious. Of course, laughter can be hurtful if not shared by all, or if a person feels he is the object of the joke. How can we promote the healing effects of humor and laughter?

The first step is to create an environment where the care partners also experience well-being, and where being joyful is considered an acceptable, even valuable part of the job. Having a good time while you work does not mean that the job is being done poorly. In fact, studies have suggested that those who have fun on the job often outperform their peers. The positive emotional landscape will carry over to the people living there, not only in creating joy, but also in cementing the relationships and regard between the elders and those who care for them.

Another ingredient is spontaneity. It is very hard to schedule joy on the activity calendar. There must be enough flexibility to go with the flow and build on a spontaneous moment. The introduction of small children or pets into a living environment is another way to create unexpected pleasures, as they are likely to be spontaneous even within a routinized activity.

Laughter also holds the seeds of hope, which helps people find meaning in adversity. In Cathy Greenblat's excellent photo essay, *Love, Loss, and Laughter: Seeing Dementia Differently*, Richard Taylor tells a story that occurred not long after his diagnosis:

On one of the first days after my diagnosis, there was a moment of absurdity in our household and I started to laugh. My wife, Linda, then started to laugh. We sat there laughing until we cried tears of joy, tears that connected us, tears that proved we were going to get through "this," whatever this was going to turn out to be. . . .

Laughter can reinforce the joy, the purposefulness, the connectedness of all human beings—if only we can see the forest of humanity instead of the trees of dementia. (p. 17)

Stimulating the Senses

Other paths to joy lead through our five senses. Sensory stimulation connects to distant memories as well as creating joy in the moment. The senses tend to be more durable than other cognitive domains in people with advanced stages of dementia (although some loss of smell can occur in some forms).

With regard to the sense of *smell*, the aroma of food cooking can reawaken dulled appetites, the smell of soil can engage a lifelong gardener, and fragrant soaps or oils can enhance the bathing experience. The olfactory centers of the brain have close connections to the memory center, and an aroma can quickly take a person back to an important moment in time and arouse old memories.

Taste can also stimulate memories and awaken one's sense of joy. While some taste treats are fairly universally enjoyed, those that have a special connection to one's past or cultural roots can be especially powerful. Holiday joy can be enhanced by the preparation of a special dish, and the food can also restore connections to home and family.

Vision may become challenged in late life, but there is still much to please even aging eyes. Simply observing children playing or the colors of autumn leaves can bring a sense of peace. Many organizations engage people living with dementia in the fine arts. The group ARTZ (Artists for Alzheimer's), founded by Dr. John Zeisel and Sean Caulfield, creates opportunities for people with dementia to attend some of the world's great museums, such as New York's MoMA, the Louvre in Paris, and Melbourne's National Gallery of Art. Greenblat's photobook chronicles a trip to the Louvre made by a group of people living with Alzheimer's, sitting with rapt expressions as they behold the masterpieces.

Sound has been described in detail for its potential to create anxiety in people living with cognitive disorders, but it can also be a source of comfort, meaning, and even growth. As described in Chapter 4, the Music and Memory project has not only re-engaged people who had been noncommunicative, but has also improved their abilities to retrieve memories and share them with others. Music can improve one's mood and create moments of peaceful contemplation or energetic participation. Of course, the music choices need to provide a personal, meaningful connection to be of greatest benefit.

Ann Davidson (1997), in her memoir of caring for her husband, Julian, a former physiology professor at Stanford Medical School, describes his ardent love of classical music. He continued to attend concerts and sing in a choir for as long as he was able. Near the close of her narrative, she describes a day when, "wearing earphones and listening to Vivaldi, he waved his arms wildly about, 'conducting' the entire *Four Seasons . . .* immersed in pleasure" (p. 223).

In going about our daily duties, we often underestimate the power of *touch*. In an environment where physical contact occurs too seldom (and is often cold or clinical when it does occur), touching with tender intent can create feelings of security as well as connectedness and joy. Lustbader (1991) interviewed a woman who had been hospitalized for eye surgery. Although her sight was impaired, she had a durable memory of one special nurse:

> I knew the nurses by their hands. There was one with such delicate fingers that I cried a little when I heard her come on duty. She made me feel like she had all the time in the world. The others made me feel like a lump of flesh, like they had to get me out of the way as fast as they could. But those hands! . . . You can't imagine how it felt to me in that strange place, to be touched like that." (pp. 52–53)

This story reminds us that the intent behind the touch is what makes the difference. It is not enough to simply go through the motions. Professionals who practice massage or therapeutic touch report that people living with dementia often relax or speak more fluently during or after a session.

Finally, the various senses can be combined, an example being an aromatic bubble bath with soft music playing. There is no limit to the ways in which we can connect the first six domains through the senses to create joy.

When speaking at St. John's Home in 2011, Taylor stated, "I don't believe people lose memories with Alzheimer's so much as they lose the ability to access those memories. Otherwise, how do you explain a person who suddenly has a day when they remember a lot of things they had previously forgotten? Those memories were always there—they just needed a key to unlock them."

The five senses provide such a key. The literature is full of stories of people who responded to some combination of sensory stimulation that opened a "back door" to engagement. Taylor (2011) also told of being interviewed on the telephone by a writer who decided to place the call from his mother's room at the nursing home during a visit he and his family had scheduled. He used her speakerphone to conduct the interview.

The interview went on for some time, when suddenly Taylor heard what sounded like crying on the other end of the line. Afraid that he had said something to upset someone, he asked what was wrong. The family had become overwhelmed because their mother, who had not spoken in months, looked at the phone and said, "That man knows what he is talking about."

Joy in Quiet Moments

In a task-centered culture of care, we often forget that joy can exist in those spaces where no apparent activity is taking place. Quiet reflection can bring us moments of contentment, as can passively observing the world around us. Many of the experiences that stimulate the five senses are also very much "being" moments, because the most important effect they have is internal—the engagement of memory, connection, emotion, or introspection that is triggered.

> It is in this solitude that we discover that being is more important than having, and that we are worth more than the result of our efforts. In solitude we discover that our life is not a possession to be defended, but a gift to be shared. (Nouwen, 2004, p.26)

In Chapter 1, we talked about the attention to detail that can occur when one moves "beyond the tyranny of time." DeBaggio (2002), who operated a nursery for much of his career, comments on his appreciation of the experiences he had previously passed over, and their restoration of his faith in the continuation of life:

> I have grown to enjoy the surprises of everyday life and self-discovery it brings. I cling to dirt and watch marvels rise from it. I watch the robin high up in the unused greenhouse, patiently warming her five

blue eggs in the fuzz of her feathers. I wait as anxiously as she to see new life. Dreams do not die even in the face of death. (p. 201)

Shouse (2006) observes the meaning of quiet moments with her mother, even when she was unable to participate in many activities:

> I sink into my mother's face like she is a meditation. We smile at each other for a half-hour, something we have never done before, something that would be too intense, too personal in our earlier, rational life together. (p. 125)

This shows once again the pleasure that such moments create for both the person with dementia and her loved one. In a similar vein, Wong (2009) found that such small pleasures created some of the most durable memories of his mother in the last years of his life—memories that showed him that life with Alzheimer's did not have to be a life of pure tragedy:

> It started out the worst of times, but ended up better than she could ever have imagined. Alzheimer's knew no mercy, yet gave my mother the happiest two years of her life.
>
> If not for Alzheimer's, routine ways would have persisted. Ma and I would not have exchanged so many "I love you"s [sic] . . .
>
> If not for Alzheimer's we would not have talked about ordinary things, enjoyed simple pleasures, sucked durian seeds together. In the slowness of Alzheimer's time, we prayed for each other, shared our thoughts, and expressed whatever stirred our hearts. (p. 3–4)

As an aside, I met Mr. Wong while speaking in Singapore, and I have also sampled durian fruit. It is definitely an acquired taste. In fact, the odor of the fruit (which resembles that of rotting flesh) is so pungent that the open fruit is banned from all public transport in Singapore. Durian would not bring *me* joy, a reminder that simple pleasures must always be individualized.

As the preceding quotes illustrate, the letting go associated with falling into forgetfulness can create space and freedom for the care partner as well, and provide a lasting lesson about the value of life. At the close of the novel *The Madonnas of Leningrad* (Dean, 2007), a young man recounts meeting Marina after she wandered away, became lost, and ended up in a cabin in the woods, where he found her and returned her to her daughter, Helen:

She pulled herself to her feet and, hanging on to his arm, started kind of leading him around the perimeter of the room, stopping every couple of feet and pointing. He remembered he was worried because she was barefoot, and there were nails and wood scraps all over the floor. "Look out," he said, and she nodded, her eyes lit bright, and said, "Look."

"Look?" he repeated.

"Look," she answered, and pointed. "It is beautiful, yes?"

"What was beautiful?" Helen had asked the young man, puzzled.

"Everything, man. That's what was so amazing. There's a killer view of the straits, but she was pointing at everything, you know, the dead madrona tree out back, and these bands of sunlight coming through the roof in the garage." Here, the young man's expression had turned very earnest. "It was like she was saying everything was beautiful."

The doctor said Marina was in shock, but Helen has always preferred the young man's explanation. "You had to be there," he insisted, "She was showing me the world." (pp. 227–228)

Faith, Spirituality, and Essence

For those with a strong faith tradition, engaging in the practice of that faith is a source of great joy and comfort. This can be attained through prayer, music, or simply sharing the experience of a quiet, meditative environment. Others may find their spirituality in nature—the sound of birds or the splashing of water in a stream. Knowing what soothes each person's soul can create joy that sustains people through more difficult moments.

Once, while working at St. John's Home, I walked past their lovely chapel. Often, when there is no service in progress, the lights are dimmed and soft music is broadcast, creating a meditative space for staff and elders alike. I glanced in and saw one of our former recreation therapists, Mary Ann, sitting quietly with three women who lived with advanced dementia. Each woman was calm and contemplative, and each face held an expression of utter contentment.

It turned out that the afternoon had been a particularly stressful one in their living area; nerves were frazzled and tempers were high. Mary Ann had decided that the chapel might give these three a respite from the commotion, and in doing so, she restored a sense of balance and security to them at a particularly difficult time.

For many who have lost the ability to converse, such quiet moments can hold the same power as a stimulating conversation or a meaningful activity. For those who are largely unable to connect in other ways, there is often an essence that maintains an important connection with those who can stop and embrace the meaning of being in the moment. In recalling his trips to visit a friend with advanced dementia, DeBaggio (2002), observes that "when the words and memories dropped away, her essence became more pronounced and delightful" (p. 152).

An Example of Seven Domains Combined

I will close this chapter with a story that nicely demonstrates the confluence of the seven domains in the context of an interaction I had with a gentleman, "Martin," when I worked at St. John's Home. I was asked by the staff at the nursing home to stop by and see him because they found it very difficult to care for him, and they were looking for suggestions.

He was often resistive to their attempts to provide personal care; he would shout, swear, and sometimes try to bite or strike out at the staff. He did not partake of activities and preferred to eat his meals alone in his room with the television on. The staff reported that, during a period of several weeks when his wife was staying at the nursing home for rehabilitation, he had been quite happy and pleasant, but since she had returned home "he has been really nasty."

Martin was not a total stranger to me. He had family members working at the home and he was known for his booming baritone voice and his love of singing. A couple of years earlier, we had enlisted him to join our annual Christmas caroling group, and he accompanied us around the home, adding his sonorous voice. But since that time, his cognitive abilities had declined and he had withdrawn to his room.

I stopped by to visit Martin. He was eating his lunch in his bedroom, as usual. I reintroduced myself and asked if he would like me to visit. He seemed very happy to have me sit and talk with him.

I asked Martin some general questions about how he was feeling and how things were going for him at the home. Initially, his answers were pleasant and positive, but somewhat superficial. After a few minutes, I probed a bit deeper, asking if he had any difficulties. At that point he acknowledged that the staff were having difficulties with *him*.

I asked Martin when those difficulties occurred and he said, "When I get nasty." I asked if he could tell me why he felt nasty, and he replied, "Because of all this," gesturing with his hands to encompass himself, sitting in a nursing home chair with a tray of food in front of him. The meaning of the gesture was obvious: he had never expected to spend the last days of his life this way.

He continued to speak quietly: "I never needed anybody's help before. I was always able to do for myself. I looked after my wife; now I can't do anything." I asked what gave him pleasure; he mentioned his wife and told me how much he missed her and wanted to be close to her. I asked him about music, and he agreed that this had also been a source of great joy in the past, but seemed to indicate that it was no longer available to him.

He told me he had been active in his church and loved to sing all the old hymns and gospel tunes. I told him I knew a few of those tunes and could play the piano a bit. I asked if he would be interested in sharing some songs with me after lunch. He politely declined and seemed unwilling or unable to contemplate moving out of his chair to the lounge area where the piano sat. I asked if he might consider sharing music later in the afternoon. He was somewhat noncommittal, so I suggested he think it over and told him I would be back in a couple of hours.

When I returned, he was still sitting in his chair with the television on. I asked again if he would like to sing some songs. He indicated that he did not really think he could sing anymore, but with some gentle prodding, I was able to convince him to come out and listen while I attempted a few of his favorite old songs.

I set Martin up beside the piano and found a few books of hymns and spirituals, possibly left there by his family. Although not extensively schooled in piano, I have the ability to play songs I know by ear with passable technique. I was surprised to find that many of the hymns in the book were familiar to me from childhood, and began to work my way through those tunes.

Martin closed his eyes with a pleasurable look on his face as I played the tunes. He would occasionally hum a few of the notes tentatively, as if testing to see if he still had a voice. He began to request songs, and if I recognized them, I played them. He soon began to forget his self-consciousness and sang out more fully, and his deep sonorous voice returned, as did the words.

After some time, we turned the page to "Amazing Grace." I know the tune well and was able to embellish a bit more as I played it. He sang, but not quite as forcefully as he had on some of the other songs. My singing along did not change that. I recall feeling a bit disappointed that he was not opening up more to this favorite hymn.

Then, after I stopped playing the song, Martin leaned forward and said, "Now, you have to learn to phrase it the way we sing it. Listen to me." He then began to sing a cappella, abandoning the waltz rhythm for a much more soulful phrasing true to his gospel tradition. I returned to the keyboard, and as I played along, he sang, conducted, and spoke directions to me, showing me exactly the proper feel and phrasing of the hymn as he had learned it in the African-American tradition.

In the space of about a half hour, Martin had become the teacher. He was animated, taking charge, telling me exactly how I should express the soulful joy of the song, and singing now in full voice. Staff members would occasionally stop as they passed by, smile, and say, "Martin, it is so good to see you out of your room and enjoying the music!" When he returned to his room after our session, he looked like a new man—confident, engaged, and filled with a peaceful spirit.

So what is the lesson from this story? Other staff members could easily say that they do not have the time I spent engaging him in song. They could also say that they do not have my exceptional ear, or even my less-than-exceptional piano technique. So how could this help them in their daily interactions?

But as I later explained to one co-worker, the true magic did not reside in the singing of songs. That was the end result of an interaction that tapped into all aspects of well-being and started before we came to the piano. The real magic was getting Martin to agree to come out of the room and engage in the music in the first place.

It began with identity and connectedness, a conversation about who he was, what he was experiencing, and the effects of his separation from the woman he loved. My suggestion to share some music was initially declined, and it was clear that he also felt that he had little control in his surroundings, which made him insecure and unsure of himself.

My response was to try to restore some security and autonomy. I spent time helping him feel comfortable with me and gave him space to express his feelings, lending a nonjudgmental ear. I then gave him some time to consider my request, and the ability to decide upon my return whether he wanted to join me or not. In doing these things, the stage was set for him to be willing to come out of the room and be engaged. The power and meaning of the music did the rest; he was able to reconnect with a great source of joy, and experienced almost immediate growth, regaining his voice and his ability to teach me and to direct the remainder of the activity.

The last part could have been re-created by simply sharing a recording of favorite songs with him. My ability to play piano was not the key; by the time he approached the lounge, the path to restoring well-being was laid. And a man living with significant dementia taught a former Eastman School jazz student how to play "Amazing Grace."

CHAPTER 10

The Experiential Pathway to Well-Being

A Well-Being Approach

The task of leadership is to create an alignment of
strengths, making our weaknesses irrelevant.

—Peter Drucker

Difficulties can be transcended. There is always a new way.
The choice is ours.

—Lela Knox Shanks

Once you can accept the universe as matter expanding
into nothing that is something, wearing stripes with plaid
comes easy.

—Albert Einstein

I HAVE JUST DEVOTED many pages to exploring a framework of seven
domains of well-being. The discussion was meant to be both broad and
deep, but it is far from complete. The paths to each aspect of well-being
are as numerous as the people living with dementia and all of their
care partners. My intent was to provide sufficient examples for each
domain so that this framework could be understood and applied to the
individuals in your care.

Let us pause and reflect for a moment. The format of this book
may be challenging to many readers, as it does not follow a traditional
structure. I did this for two reasons. First, I wanted to shake readers out
of the orderly path in order to help you break out of traditional ways of

thinking about this collection of shifting experiences we have come to label "dementia." In this way, I intended to share a bit of the nonlinear thinking that people living with the condition often experience, as well as to open your minds to creative ideas that do not reveal themselves in a more traditional format.

More important, however, was my desire to shift your thinking to a view firmly centered on well-being. In order for this chapter to have a maximum impact, it is important to let go of a deficit-based approach to supporting people living with changing cognitive abilities and move to a strength-based, proactive approach.

I have been teaching this approach in my seminars and have noticed that it is very difficult for participants to break out of the old mindset. But when they do, it provides valuable insights that had been invisible to them up to that point.

As I mentioned at the beginning of the book, our most common blind spot—even among person-centered care advocates—involves seeing the distress as the problem, rather than a symptom of a larger need. And the need is usually larger than we realize; even when we identify a simple need that has not been met, fulfilling that need may not be enough if there are severe losses in several areas of well-being.

Furthermore, when we are unable to identify a specific need or trigger, we usually fall back either on the use of psychotropic medications or on the continued use of interventions that may divert but not prevent the underlying distress from recurring. This is why we need to go much deeper in order to have a more profound effect on the lives of people living with dementia.

The key, I believe, is right here in well-being. I believe that erosion of well-being is at the root of the vast majority of episodes of ill-being that are experienced by a person living with dementia. This is why I have dedicated so much space to dissecting these seven domains, examining the forces that erode them and the ways in which we can restore them through transformative approaches.

In my years of practice, I have learned how our focus on disease and deficits has held us back in understanding how best to provide support for people in all living environments, while simultaneously creating barriers to self-fulfillment for those individuals. The result of my efforts has been to reframe dementia using a model that puts the experience of the person at the center. In doing so, it became clear to me what each person living with changing cognition needs most, and that is to experience the same opportunities for well-being that each of us desires.

In setting forth these ideas, I have chosen one framework for understanding well-being that resonates with me and whose components are easily accessible to a wide audience. This approach has helped me to examine many aspects of daily life and care with a critical eye and to find new insights to share. As I described in Chapter 2, there are numerous legitimate models that outline a pathway to well-being, and one could have built a similar book around any of them. But beyond the choice of a particular model, the true value of a well-being approach lies in the *process* that I will now describe. I call this approach the Experiential Pathway to Well-Being. Those who prefer a different set of domains are invited to use the format of the preceding seven chapters, as well as the approach I am about to outline, substituting their preferred model. My guess is that any good model for well-being will be equally successful when applied in the manner I am describing.

A graphic representation of the Experiential Pathway to Well-Being model is shown in Figure 4. It represents a more dynamic interpretation of the well-being pyramid illustrated in Chapter 5. In this

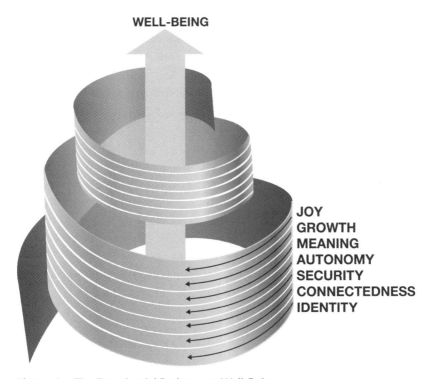

Figure 4. The Experiential Pathway to Well-Being.

new image, the seven domains not only build on each other to promote increasing levels of well-being, but they also represent our metaphoric *ramps*, providing gateways for continuously feeding the essential components of well-being into a person's day-to-day existence.

The Experiential Pathway to Well-Being can be used in two ways. First, it should create a process for supporting the person living with dementia on an ongoing basis by understanding how her well-being is challenged and then striving to restore as much of each aspect as possible. But setting a primary goal of well-being also provides a very useful mindset for decoding distress, and finds answers to unmet needs that other approaches fail to provide.

I rattle my cage but no one comes to feed me. (DeBaggio, 2002, p. 185)

Using the Experiential Pathway to Understand Distress

In *Dementia Beyond Drugs*, I described an approach to understanding distress that involves three "audits." The medical audit looks for physical illness, pain, or medication effects that could underlie such distress. The environmental audit looks at attributes of the environment (noise, temperature, food/drink/bowel/bladder needs, etc.) that could be triggers. Most of these potential causes of distress are well known to care partners and are extensively taught in other approaches.

The third audit is the *experiential audit*, which looks at distress as unmet needs and strives to understand the experience of the person behind the expression. This framework still applies when using the Experiential Pathway to Well-Being, because medical and environmental problems should always be identified and addressed when present.

However, I believe that the first two categories account for only a small proportion of the distress we see on a day-to-day basis. The experiential audit is the level at which most care partners get stuck. This explains why the recurrence of daily distress and the ongoing use of medications continue to be significant in all living environments. Furthermore, understanding the unique experience and needs of the person can be a difficult task, especially if the person has trouble verbally expressing himself or is severely impaired in other cognitive areas.

These are the people for whom the Experiential Pathway to Well-Being is especially useful in opening new doors to understanding. Here is how it works:

1. *Assemble the care partner team.* The first step is to bring together all those who partner in care and who have knowledge of the person and insights to share. It should be emphasized that those with the most proximity to the person have an important contribution regardless of job title, and should have a central role in leading the discussion. In the nursing home, this not only includes hands-on staff, but possibly others who spend time with the person, such as a housekeeper or a volunteer. In the community, it could be a close neighbor, a home health worker, or the person who drives the van to a day center.

2. *Record your observations.* The second step is to describe the observed expressions fully and *nonjudgmentally*—their frequency, setting, what they look like; alleviating factors; and other characteristics. (It may be helpful to review the interventions that have been tried to date, but as I stated in the Prologue, these usually do not get to the heart of the issue, which is why the person has been brought to the discussion in the first place.)

3. *Ensure the person is well known.* When I am consulted about a challenging situation, I always try to begin by asking what people know about the *person*, and it is striking how often very little is known beyond the name, medical history, immediate relations, and ongoing care needs. So as care partners move forward, they need to generate a more thorough personal and relational history in order to maximize their ability to restore well-being (remember that the first domain we explored was *identity*).

4. *Look through the person's eyes.* Step four requires a concerted effort in order to step out of our own reality and try to see what the person sees and feel what he feels. Different forms of role-play can be very helpful at this stage. Once again, the task is not to judge whether the person's expressions have merit, nor even necessarily to understand them, but to experience them as fully as possible.

5. *Turn your focus to well-being.* This is where the insights usually appear, but it is also the hardest step by far. The support team needs to put their discussion of the distress completely aside, then simply

look at each domain of well-being and begin to craft a plan to rebuild each domain for the person over time. With large groups, this can be done by breaking into seven teams, or with smaller groups by exploring the domains one at a time.

Why is this such a hard step? Because we become stuck in the mindset of "fixing the behavior." As a result, the team will have a tendency to fall back into problem-solving mode. That is a reactive and deficit-based approach; if it worked, the person's problem would have been solved long ago.

Therefore, the key to this approach (using the disability metaphor) is to *turn our backs on the "behavior," and find the "ramps" to improved well-being.* What will result are seven lists of proactive, strength-based approaches that can enhance each domain of well-being and restore a sense of balance for a person who is living in a very unbalanced world. And if done correctly, these lists will contain a wealth of information that the previous problem-based approach did not identify or address. As suggested by the previous chapters, these approaches will overlap and feed into each other, as no aspect of well-being exists independently.

There is an important caveat here: this approach rarely supplies a quick fix to these complex issues. If there were a quick fix, the problem would have resolved and not recurred. Also, we discussed that each domain of well-being is enhanced through personal, operational, and physical transformations; these are multifaceted, organic processes that can take time to implement, especially in living environments that are still very institutional. What it provides, however, is a pathway to long-term, sustainable success. Remember, too, that supporting well-being is a never-ending journey, as each of our life circumstances, relationships, and abilities continue to shift throughout our lives.

Many homes in the United States have already lowered their antipsychotic use by 15% or more since the federal initiative began in 2012. The problem is that many of these gains may be the result of quick-fix interventions, and, therefore, may be short-lived if a foundation for long-term well-being is not established. I believe the Experiential Pathway to Well-Being will enable organizations to reduce medication use to a bare minimum, and keep it there.

Teaching the Experiential Pathway to Well-Being

In my in-depth workshops, I often lead the class through this approach, using a real-life situation that one of the participants shares. For teaching purposes, it is best to start with a well-circumscribed story involving a person who is fairly familiar to the presenter of the case. These guidelines are helpful because (1) it is best not to waste an hour of the exercise telling a long and convoluted story, and (2) the person presenting the story should know enough about the person in question to supply answers to any basic background questions the group might pose.

A frequent observation that is quite telling is that many of the class's follow-up questions to the presenter revolve around a litany of "Have you tried (this or that intervention)?" Such is our usual mindset of trying to fix the behavior we see.

Once we have spent some time getting a basic story and background information on the person, we break into seven teams—one assigned to each well-being domain. Each team is asked to use the information they have gained, but to put the behavioral expression completely aside and simply generate a list of ways in which they might enhance their assigned domain of well-being for this particular person. Of course, the class cannot possibly know this person well enough to find all of the keys to his individual well-being. But they have all seen people with similar challenges, and the point of the exercise is not necessarily to solve one particular real-life challenge but to teach the thought process that they will then use when they meet to discuss people they support and know well.

This approach requires a lot of coaching, so deeply ingrained is our tendency to favor reactive interventions—to try and fix the "cough" (expression of distress) rather than the "pneumonia" (deeper well-being needs). I often find I have to walk around to the various lists and point out which items are only addressing the cough versus the pneumonia, until the participants begin to adopt the proper mindset.

Before setting the class to work on their individual lists, I ask each team to begin by imagining that their assigned well-being domain is a drinking glass that is somewhere between being totally empty and totally full. They should ask themselves, "Based on what we have heard, how full is this person's 'identity glass' at present?" Or, "How full is his 'connectedness glass?'" and so on for each of the seven domains. They should then draw the glass at the top of their poster, with the level of well-being indicated.

When this exercise is done well, two powerful insights emerge. The first insight occurs when we look at their seven drawings of drinking glasses representing the domains of well-being. Keep in mind that most nursing home employees are talented, compassionate people, and when the class asks what interventions they have tried, it becomes clear that they have usually tried nearly every approach that the group can suggest. But when the drawings are shared, it is unusual to find any glass more than 25% full, and many are shown to be nearly empty. In other words, even though these talented care partners have tried every intervention they know, we have identified seven areas of need that their current approach did not even begin to address! This shows the limitations of a problem-based approach.

The second insight emerges from sharing the well-being lists. Once again, even though the person may not be familiar to most of the participants, lists are generated that contain ideas that our reactive approach never considered. These ideas were invisible, partly because they do not directly respond to the "behavior," and also because they focus on creating an *infrastructure* for long-term wellness.

Our time-and-task mentality is such that approaches that do not appear to directly attack the challenge are not considered or valued. Yet if erosion of these domains is the root cause of the distress, then our ultimate goal is to address these, if we are ever to succeed.

This exercise is much more difficult than it looks on paper; we are deeply buried within the paradigm of the biomedical model. Sometimes the case presented in the class is not a great starting case for the uninitiated, or sets the bar too high for novices to this approach. Sometimes, the class has not been able to shift their paradigm enough to truly optimize the process. But once the insights appear to the group, the results are so dramatic that I have seen the case presenters pull the various flip charts off of the easels and enthusiastically package them up for their colleagues back at their nursing home, saying, "There is so much we can be doing that never occurred to us!"

Many class participants have written later to say that they began using this approach in their team meetings, and a new world of solutions has begun to appear. This is the power of the Experiential Pathway to Well-Being.

As with learning any new skill, it is probably best not to start with your most challenging situation. Begin with those whose expressions are less complex or more predictable, and for whom you can easily obtain more background information from family and friends. You do not learn how to do the high jump by starting with the bar set at 6 feet.

Often, it is evident that one or two domains are especially affected by a situation. For example, many cases of people being resistive or physically reactive during care primarily involve the domain of autonomy, and possibly security as well. Therefore, it is possible to prioritize the domains you explore and your resultant approaches, in order to get more traction early on.

Even in situations such as those described above, all seven domains are probably involved to some extent; such is the nature of the challenges to personhood created both by the illness and by our traditional approach to care. But, because a successful approach must address several fronts over a period of time, it can be useful to start with the ones that will have the greatest effect in the short run, so that initial improvements in the person's well-being can propel the initiatives forward and bring early relief for all.

In the case of physical reactivity, the team might start by restoring autonomy in as many ways as possible, with a secondary view toward enhancing security. As this initiative rolls out, the team can then look at aspects of the other domains to bring into play—enhancing the person's identity, firming up connections, or adding meaning by ritualizing his daily routine, to name a few examples.

You may recall that the preceding seven chapters described ways in which each aspect of well-being can be enhanced through personal, operational, and physical transformation. Each successful approach usually requires a fundamental change of attitude, and perhaps changes to the physical environment as well; but I believe the key to sustained success will most often lie in the *operational* transformation. This applies to organizations as well as individuals supporting a person in her own home. When the systems and routines around daily life can successfully shift and better support the individual's needs, desires, and abilities, it becomes easier to shift them further as those needs, desires, and abilities change; and in congregate living environments, the operational shifts make it easier to accommodate more individual needs as they arise, with less disruption or dismantling of the overall system of care over time.

Applying the Experiential Pathway to Well-Being: A Real-Life Example

I was once asked to offer advice to staff members caring for "Dorothy," a woman living with dementia who had recently moved to their neighborhood at the nursing home. This move had capped a series of relocations that had happened in relatively short order. Only a few months before she had lived at home with her husband, who was her "rock" and who had provided support for her through her cognitive changes.

Her husband's death led to Dorothy being moved to an assisted living home; but because of increasing care needs, she soon was transferred to St. John's Home. Unfortunately, a renovation plan at the home led to her being uprooted once again and moved to her current room.

Dorothy was a strong "family" person. She stayed home with her children while they were young, and provided them with a lot of structure and practical advice in their formative years. After the children were grown, she worked in various jobs—as a waitress, a cleaner, and a secretary. Her family described her as being very "down to earth" and possessing a strong work ethic. She was also an "independent thinker" who "never followed the crowd." She loved music (especially Frank Sinatra, Bobby Darin, and various show tunes), Italian food, and chocolate.

The group asked me to help them address several issues that arose during her daily life on the neighborhood. Dorothy would frequently call out loudly. Sometimes this was related to specific requests (food, drink, toilet); at other times she would call out the names of family members, or simply reach out and try to grab hold of those in her vicinity.

Dorothy was often soothed by a gentle, tender touch, such as stroking her cheek. However, during personal care, she would often grab the care partner's arm and dig in with her nails. There were rare instances of her attempting to strike at or even bite the care partner.

She was seen to be "impulsive," in that her care partners could not identify a pattern or obvious trigger to these expressions. Often, when staff members tried to intervene, she became more distressed or resistive, and they learned that the best response at these times was to back off.

Dorothy's ability to walk was hampered by both a general unsteadiness on her feet and a tendency to see shiny floors as being wet. She made frequent attempts to stand, which were often interrupted with attempts to re-seat her. She had been prescribed psychoactive medications for her distress; these only resulted in brief periods of quiet at best, and "as needed" doses were variously reported as effective or ineffective in her record.

An initial "looking through her eyes" exercise helped the group to identify a number of losses—her husband, her home of 50 years, her regular contact with family members, and her independence. It was suggested that she might have unresolved grief, since she was uprooted so quickly after the death of her husband, her "rock."

The care partners were also able to imagine that she might have feelings of both frustration and fear in her present situation, and that loss of control could be contributing to those feelings.

Two possible medical contributors that were raised were hearing loss and persistent pain from a fractured pelvis two months prior; but her ear examination was normal and she appeared to move without pain when assisted.

An examination of Dorothy's strengths revealed that she was able to state her desires clearly on at least some occasions, and that she responded to her name, though no one was clear if she responded best to "Dorothy," "Mrs. G.," or "Do" (the pet name her husband had used). She could converse readily at times, but became fatigued if presented with too many questions. Dorothy's love of music, food, and chocolate were identified as strengths, as was her ability to be loving and affectionate at times.

In this instance, the focus on time and task had caused the care partners to forget many of the basic "face-to-face" communication and facilitation skills that I discussed in my first book, so these were reiterated. It seemed possible that the worsening of her distress with attempted interventions might be largely due to the manner in which she was being approached. Attention to these interactions was able to improve their response to some extent, but there was little change in the overall situation.

The above scenario is typical of many challenges faced by caring staff. Their focus on how best to respond to her words and actions led to an impasse in which her care partners only occasionally felt they were answering her needs, and often were perplexed by what appeared to be impulsive behavior. This is a perfect place to begin crafting a well-being approach.

By focusing on domains of well-being, rather than responses to distress, a new plan can be adopted that will lead to far better success in the long run. I coached the group through this approach, and while the examples listed below are not exhaustive, they will illustrate how this approach leads to new insights.

Using the Seven Domains to Create a Well-Being Plan

Using the glass full–empty analogy, the *identity* well-being domain probably fares the best of the seven, though there is still much to be done. Dorothy's "identity glass" is about 50% full at best. Part of the approach involves discovering more about her basic identity—how she prefers to be addressed, about her home of 50 years, and what she values most about her past life.

The other part of identity involves understanding how it is evolving and how to support this in her new living environment. The sudden loss of husband and home no doubt has left some unresolved grief. Use of "transitional objects"—important objects or mementos from her past life to help create a bridge to her new life—can be very comforting, and may also be an aid to helping her express her grief more fully.

Using our knowledge of Dorothy—favorite foods, music, past work—we can also begin to build a relationship and rapport by asking about these and referring to them in daily discourse and activities. The key in building identity is to go beyond simply recognizing her history and understand her need to form a durable identity within her new surroundings.

The level of her *connectedness* domain was felt to be very low for Dorothy—less than 20%. This is evident, not only in her history of bereavement and frequent moves, but also in her frequent calling out, reaching out, and grabbing onto care partners and passersby. While there are largely dedicated staff assignments at St. John's Home, this is a case where connectedness is critical, and every effort should be taken to preserve those primary relationships and minimize the number of people who provide hands-on assistance (and whose identity must be learned by her).

We can use the information gleaned about her identity to connect her to those favorite foods, music, and love of family within her new living space by engaging her with these—through conversation or focused activities around cooking and meal planning, music appreciation, or planning holiday celebrations and family events. All of the facilitative skills that enable communication and working through tasks that were described in Chapter 4 will also improve the success of such engagement.

The use of personalized music might be particularly beneficial here, since her tastes are so well known. However, this is not something that should just be applied indiscriminately during the day, as staff desire. Instead, they should offer her music at various times and engage her with it as she listens, in order to better understand what her connection is to the songs and when music might be most beneficial for her.

As also described in Chapter 4, the staff should take time and effort to stop and visit with her for a few minutes on regular occasions, unrelated to scheduled tasks or to instances of her calling out. During these times, they should share their presence with her, perhaps adding conversation and/or gentle touch as able. By increasing her familiarity with them, they can also help her feel that she belongs in this space, has a meaningful relationship with those around her, and does not need to call out to warrant personal attention.

The level of Dorothy's *security* domain is also very low—less than 20%. Her frequent actions of calling out and reaching for people indicate a need for reassurance and the security of connection, so the approach mentioned in the previous paragraph will help enhance security as well. The frequent moves, none of which were within her control, have also eroded her security, so attention to bridging identity and stability in the new living environment will help her to feel more settled.

Dorothy's visual interpretation of the floors as being wet is another threat to security, one which might make her attempts to walk even more risky, due to her anxiety about the surface on which she is stepping. This is a common phenomenon when people living with cognitive change encounter high-glare surfaces. Use of low-gloss cleaning products and reduced polishing provides a better surface for walking. (Despite what we were told by 1960s television ads, a sense of security is more important than shiny floors.)

As a person who was an "independent thinker" who "never followed the crowd," Dorothy's level of *autonomy* is likely to be nearly nonexistent in an environment where she is redirected every time she attempts to stand, and is otherwise subject to schedules and routines set by others. To the extent to which she is offered generic group activities, her ability to be a nonconformist is also squelched. While her *ability* to do for herself and follow her own muse may be compromised, her inner nature to do so is likely still very strong, and must be recognized.

To that point, every interaction needs to seek her input and direction to the extent she is able. She should be engaged in conversation about her values and desires, so that her care partners can understand those traits that make her unique. Her well-being plan needs to reflect that uniqueness in each part of her daily life, from the way in which she enjoys her meals to the order in which her morning routine proceeds.

Dorothy is able to walk with assistance, and so her attempts to stand should engage both some guided physical activity (to relieve her restlessness and boredom) and critical thinking about what else her attempts to stand might signify. While this will take some staff adjustment at the outset, a proactive effort to meet the needs behind her attempts to walk will better reflect her individuality and personal rhythms, produce marked improvements in her level of restlessness, and likely improve her strength and balance as well.

In Dorothy's case, the first four domains also have a close connection to the domains of *meaning* and *growth*; once again, the current levels of these two domains are very low, probably less than 10%. So in this category, some key questions to consider might include the following: How can we create more meaning for an "independent thinker" through enhancing her individuality and autonomy? How can we take our knowledge of her past history to create more daily opportunities for meaning and purpose? What would bring meaning to the life of a person who was a primary family support, a secretarial assistant, a cleaner, or a waitress? How does a person with these personal and professional backgrounds feel when she constantly sees floors that appear to be wet? How does a person who spent her life engaged in assisting others, providing stability in home and work, and lending her expertise continue to find meaning and growth through caregiving and mentoring opportunities in her present life?

Examination of these questions will lead to a better understanding of ways in which Dorothy can continue to be useful and contribute to the life of her new home. The restoration of meaningful rituals and roles in her daily life will help her to regain her sense of control, her sense of self-worth, and a new sense of "home" in her new surroundings that gets to the heart of her distress. She can also share her interests with staff and elders alike, regaining her identity as a person with wisdom and experience to dispense.

Dorothy's sense of *joy*, which is intermittent at best, can be better sustained when the above domains are addressed; but it can also be enhanced in the short term by creating simple pleasures based on those that have already been identified. These include her love of certain kinds of music, of good food, of tender touch, and of family. Such pleasures can be enjoyed spontaneously and individually, but can also be combined, such as the use of favorite music, aromatic soaps, and affectionate touch, to create a spa-like bathing experience. Once again, such approaches must not simply be generated as a "laundry list" of ideas that *we* think might work, but instead should flow from an understanding of her unique rhythms and preferences, which only a close relational approach can truly identify.

The above examples are a bit simplified—by enlisting a team of people who have come to know Dorothy well, a deeper list of approaches to well-being can be constructed. As mentioned previously in my outline of the process described above, there are two important points to take away from this example. First is that in spite of kind attention by talented and caring staff, Dorothy's distress continued, and looking at her life through a well-being lens highlighted seven areas in which her "glass" was no more than half full, and nearly empty in most instances despite their best efforts.

The second point is that the list of suggestions for improving well-being—even a bit abbreviated in this example—nevertheless shows a number of steps that are not envisioned in our typical approach to distress. This is why the staff's best efforts to help Dorothy fell short of providing any long-term improvement.

It is important to reiterate that this approach is not a quick fix for problems that have become severely ingrained over time. However, it is a far better path to durable solutions, creating an infrastructure for well-being that will shape Dorothy's future life at the home, and hopefully adapting to her needs as her life and abilities evolve. And there will never be a medication that fulfills any of the needs we have identified.

Using the Experiential Pathway to Well-Being for More Emergent Needs

The Experiential Pathway to Well-Being, therefore, is both an infrastructure for living that supports long-term wellness, as well as a tool for understanding and addressing ill-being. Seeing distress as *ill-being* (the opposite of well-being) helps move us away from the narrow biomedical view of "behaviors."

But this approach also gives insights to more emergent situations. In the past few years, as I have learned to trade in well-being, I have begun to start with this reference point whenever a challenging situation is presented to me. The following is an example of how this has helped me overcome more emergent barriers to care:

> A few years ago, I was called on a Monday morning and asked
> if I could assist with a woman, "Maxine," who had moved into
> the nursing home the previous Friday evening. She lived with

Alzheimer's, and the unfortunate nature of her arrival—she had been brought to the home by her family on the pretense that they were "going out," and then left there—had put the staff at a disadvantage from the moment of her arrival.

Over the weekend, Maxine had steadfastly declined to let anyone remove her clothing or assist with personal care. As a result, she had worn the same outfit for 3 days, the nurses had been unable to do a skin assessment, and her hygiene was of great concern. Her assigned physician suggested that the staff consult with me about the situation. Could I possibly help?

As I looked at Maxine's chart, I thought about her experience from the well-being perspective. She had been duped into coming here and now was being asked to submit to the ministrations of a group of strangers, and she was digging her heels in. While some degree of security and other domains were involved, it was clear to me that the crux of the matter centered on autonomy and the fact that a major decision about her life (the place where she would likely live out her remaining days) had been made without her input or knowledge.

Maxine was sitting quietly on a loveseat in the living room, watching the television, but also eyeing all of the goings on around her. I walked over, introduced myself, and asked if I might visit with her for a few minutes. She pleasantly welcomed me to sit beside her.

I began by spending several minutes asking her to tell me about herself, and finding out how she was feeling. Maxine continued to converse pleasantly and answer my questions as able. She showed no signs of suspicion or anger, but I had no doubt that if pressed to do something she did not want to do, she would speak out.

After several minutes of conversation and connection, I mentioned that I was a doctor and that I would love to take a quick listen to her heart and lungs, in the privacy of her room, to make sure she was in good health. Would she be willing to do that? She seemed unsure.

I told her that it was completely up to her, but that I would like to check her if possible. I told her I would go do some other work and come back in 10 or 15 minutes to see what she had decided. Sitting back at the nurse's station, I told the nurse manager that if Maxine agreed to come with me to her room, to please have her primary nurse and aide tag along and follow my lead.

To my delight, when I returned and asked Maxine what she had decided, she readily agreed. As we walked to the room, I told her I would bring along a couple of staff members to assist us. Upon reaching the room, I did not immediately try to get her to undress or lie down. As we stood near her bed, I simply pulled out my stethoscope and listened to her heart and lungs through her blouse, as she followed my instructions for breathing softly or deeply.

After listening for a moment, I told her, "From what I can tell, your heart and lungs sound very healthy. However, I could hear a lot better if we could remove your blouse and put a gown on. Would that be okay with you?" Once again, Maxine readily agreed. We removed her blouse and draped the gown around her and I gave another listen and pronounced her to be in good shape. I asked her if she might need to use the toilet and she said she did.

The staff then helped Maxine to the toilet, and she was very willing at that point to agree to have them remove her pants as she sat down, and to get her "a nice clean set of clothes" to put on after using the toilet. In doing so, they changed her clothes, assessed her skin, and provided some initial attention to hygiene, to be built upon in future interactions.

This is an example of a situation that arose as a result of severely eroded autonomy. Although the woman's family may have caused it, this loss was also not sufficiently appreciated or addressed by the nursing home staff. Focusing their attention on time and task exacerbated the situation, as it usually does when people try to push through care with a person who is feeling a loss of control.

Once again, there was nothing magical involved. Rather, I recognized that a few extra minutes needed to be devoted to the situation early on; in other words, we often need to slow down at the beginning in order to save time in the long run.

While many of the steps just outlined centered on restoring some choice and control to the woman, note that I did not forget the base of the well-being pyramid. I began by taking a few minutes to connect and learn more about her as a person, and in doing so also *demonstrated that I cared about her as much or more than the task I had in mind.*

Finally, it is important to emphasize that autonomy, like empowerment, is not a half-hearted initiative that you "try," but then abandon as soon as you hit a snag. It is a commitment to well-being that you must honor, working through any difficulties that emerge. I had a fair idea that she would agree to be examined, based on the way in which she was responding to my approach. But if I had returned and she had declined my request, I had to be prepared to walk away and try again some other time.

If she had declined and I had pressed forward anyway after telling her that she had a choice, I would have eroded her trust even further and made the staff's job harder in the long run. This is an important point for all of us to remember—when we press against resistance in order to "get the job done" and do not honor autonomy, we create a more difficult situation for our colleagues as well as ourselves.

Finally, note that there was not simply one request made to her. I used Greenwood's principle of "continual consent" outlined in Chapter 6, never assuming that a single "yes" meant that she was understanding and accepting of all I had in mind.

When people ask how they can help their co-workers embrace a new approach, I encourage them to take advantage of "teachable moments," such as the scenario described above. Showing is often better than telling, and the positive effects of the approach will reinforce its value.

Measuring Success

With any new approach, the question inevitably arises of how one can measure whether the approach is successful. There are many issues complicating such a question. First, as mentioned in Chapter 8, there is the larger ethical concern of whether we should have to wait for research studies before we give people humanistic care. But one can certainly argue that it would be good to have a way to tell if the approach is being applied correctly, and whether our approach is giving us the benefits we expect.

As it turns out, even such nebulous concepts as these aspects of well-being can be quantified to an extent. Several years ago, I was part of a small work group convened by The Eden Alternative® to try and create a tool for measuring these seven domains. The result of our efforts was a set of three survey tools that would measure the domains of well-being in elders, professional staff, and family members. This tool has had some initial validation and larger-scale work is being done to refine it for general use.

New tools such as this are critical to research in transformational models of care, because most of our available scales for people with dementia are deficit-based, and even some of our quality-of-life scales are more reflective of medical or functional outcomes, rather than states of well-being that can be improved in people who are chronically or progressively disabled.

There are many other observational tools in current use that are based on person-centered philosophies. In most of these, environmental and situational triggers of distress may be identified, but larger, underlying well-being domains such as those outlined above are not well addressed. An approach centered upon a well-being focus is a very different one than has been traditionally employed, and, therefore, requires a very different evaluation process.

Even with the eventual development of validated tools to measure these or similar domains, enhancing well-being is not a process that is easy to study, because it is reflective of a multifactorial, long-term pathway that requires many operational shifts to be fully realized. This is not the stuff of short-term, single-intervention, placebo-controlled trials. As long as our research funding favors designs that measure success with a biomedical or pharmaceutical yardstick, any "evidence base" will be slow in coming. It is impossible to truly evaluate approaches that reject a narrow biomedical focus if we are relying exclusively on biomedical research methodology.

So we have a "Catch-22" situation, where a well-being approach requires a learning curve of new skills and operational shifts before it can be fully successful; yet academicians, regulators, and providers alike are reluctant to sanction such initiatives until we have published evidence of success.

That should not deter us from moving forward. Those who advocate to "wait for more evidence" when the research environment is stacked against the designs needed to truly evaluate a humanistic model such as the Experiential Pathway to Well-Being are simply creating another self-fulfilling prophecy. Or as Internet business guru Clay Shirky famously stated, "Institutions will try to preserve the problem to which they are the solution."

We can take a clue, once again, from the world of physics, in which the work of theoreticians has been better valued. Many discoveries, going back to Newton's gravitational theories, were postulated and developed long before they could be experimentally proven. Einstein once remarked, "Not everything that can be counted counts, and not everything that counts can be counted."

But well-being counts. The seven domains described in this book are not only universal across cultures and abilities—they are also outcomes that can never be achieved through pharmaceutical manipulation, nor through simple "interventions." While this model is still in the early stages of practical application, those organizations that have employed the Experiential Pathway to Well-Being approach are already reporting new insights and new successes for those people for whom success seemed impossible.

CHAPTER 11

Dementia and Aging in the Twenty-first Century

Reframing (and Reclaiming) Hope

with Daniella Greenwood

> Hope is not a prognostication—it's an orientation of the spirit. . . . Hope is definitely not the same thing as optimism. It is not the conviction that something will turn out well but the certainty that something makes sense, regardless of how it turns out. . . . life is too precious a thing to permit its devaluation by living pointlessly, emptily, without meaning, without love, and, finally, without hope.
>
> —Václav Havel

IN THE PRECEDING CHAPTERS, I have discussed the current state of care and support for people living with various forms of differing cognitive ability. Using a well-being framework, I have proposed an alternative, strength-based approach that can create sustainable improvements in the lives of such people and those who care for them.

In the course of this discussion, I have raised several challenging and controversial issues, which I hope will stimulate discussion and debate. Many of these issues represent the evolution of my own thinking;

Daniella Greenwood, BHlthSci, is Strategy and Innovation Manager at Arcare Australia.

as I have worked within the well-being framework, I have come to see dementia through what might be described as more of a "postmodernist lens":

> A postmodernist lens recognises difference, contradiction and frag-
> mentation—different, contradictory and fragmented identities,
> beliefs, values, sexualities, lifestyles, cultures, worldviews, mean-
> ings, narratives—indeed any issue related to the human experience.
> (Bartlett & O'Connor, 2010, p. 33)

But what of the future? How should we view and respond to the ex-
panding demographics of older people and of people living with various forms of dementia? What are the chances of a cure? And what living options await our rapidly expanding older population?

I will use this final chapter to offer some of my personal views on these issues. In doing so, I will be outlining a vision that diverges from much of the mainstream thinking around the future of dementia and the larger issue of the global aging of our population. This vision requires that we extend the strength-based approach used throughout this book to encompass all older people—regardless of a label or diagnosis—and then extend this focus to the positive potential that already exists within our diverse communities. As we do so, a different kind of future begins to emerge—one that moves us beyond forgetfulness, beyond drug therapies, and beyond cure.

The Future of Dementia

A lot of ink has been devoted to the goal of curing Alzheimer's. Many "breakthroughs" have been announced with a great deal of fanfare, but in more than a decade no new treatment approach has reached the public. It is clear that cognitive illness is far more complex than we would like to believe.

A perfect example was announced a week before I typed these pages. A team from the United Kingdom was able to arrest the neu-
ronal damage in the brains of mice "infected" with prions (elementary particles that are even more primitive than viruses, and that cause such conditions as "mad cow disease"). The media excitedly announced that stopping the neuronal degeneration in this study was a breakthrough that could have ramifications for the treatment of illnesses such as Alzheimer's or Parkinson's disease.

This does sound truly exciting, but there is good reason to temper our enthusiasm, as there are many hurdles to clear between the success of this study and a viable treatment for people living with Alzheimer's or other brain disorders. First of all, this study was done in mouse brains, not human brains. Second, the study did not measure long-term benefits or risks. Third, the drug stopped cell degeneration due to prion infections; this is not the mechanism involved with Alzheimer's or Parkinson's, so it may be another big leap to use this technique to treat these conditions. Fourth, while the drug seemed to reverse the structural damage in the brain cells, it was not a prevention, and it is difficult to tell if what appears to be healed tissue really translates to restoration of a full range of cognition when your "patient" is a mouse. Finally, getting animal research to the point of human trials and then finding the drug to be safe and effective in older adults represent another series of big leaps.

The truth is that no one really knows yet what the causes of Alzheimer's are. I wrote that statement in the plural, because I do not personally believe that there is one root cause of Alzheimer's. I think that the changes we see in the brain are a "final common pathway" for a variety of factors that can affect the brain over a lifetime—a combination of genetic risk, lifestyle, environmental exposures, and life experiences, superimposed upon an aging body.

Whitehouse & George (2008) wrote an excellent discussion of the many hypotheses regarding the cause(s) of Alzheimer's, and I recommend reading that book for more details on all the proposed mechanisms and their proponents. Though I do not possess the researchers' expertise, my personal guess is that several of these processes are occurring in tandem as the brain ages. Despite all of the prevailing theories about the cause of Alzheimer's, from glucose metabolism to misfolded proteins, inflammatory mediators, or failure of the microcirculation, it seems more likely to me that each of these camps is merely looking at one aspect of the "elephant" that is Alzheimer's, rather than seeing the whole creature.

More important, if you look at a graph representing the incidence of Alzheimer's related to a person's age, you can see an upward curve that begins to appear in midlife and rises at an increasingly rapid rate throughout the later years of life. This is not the curve one would expect from a disease with strong genetic ties. We know that genes are a very important factor in a small minority of people with Alzheimer's, but for the vast majority, the biggest risk is clearly the number of years your brain has been alive and exposed to various influences.

In other words, Alzheimer's is an illness that is intricately tied to the aging process. It is claimed that over one-third of adults ages 85 and older have signs of Alzheimer's. At what point do we cross the line between "disease" and the consequences of living to an advanced age? As long as we continue to live long lives, will there ever be a day when people do not forget more than we think is normal? I do not think so. And while we may find drugs that slow the speed of neuronal loss, the concept of a cure becomes problematic, as it would be something akin to curing aging.

In fact, perhaps the most brilliant theory I have heard to date comes from Dr. Richard Taylor (2013) in a blog he posted. In that post (referring to the near-doubling of our life expectancy since the introduction of public health initiatives and antibiotics over the last century), Taylor concluded that maybe "our brains are way behind evolving to meet our needs . . . They haven't caught up (evolved fast enough) with the fact that they are going to have to function another 20–30 years."

Even if we could wave a magic wand and make all Alzheimer's disappear tomorrow, there would still be millions of people living with dozens of other forms of cognitive illness, whether primary dementias, such as Lewy body and frontotemporal dementia, or those secondary to other illnesses, such as Parkinson's disease, alcoholism, and multiple strokes. Are we continuing to meet their needs as well?

Does this mean I have abandoned hope? Quite the opposite. In fact, I would argue that too much focus on the cure can create false hope and negatively affect the person who is living with the illness. When the vast majority of our resources and attention are focused on the ultimate goal of cure, we diminish the aspects of care and support that are life-giving; that contribute to the well-being of those who are with us today, who will not be cured.

> There is a danger when too much emphasis and hope is [sic] placed on clinical trials and the goal of "finding a cure" that issues of quality of life may be overlooked and those people currently experiencing dementia may be left to suffer in silence. (Bartlett & O'Connor, 2010, p. 13)

Once again, I am not opposed to research to find medications that might slow the rate of neuronal damage. But there is a larger problem that stems from an inordinate focus on cure, which is an inordinate focus on fixing deficits. This deficit-based approach reinforces the notion that frailty and difference should not be tolerated, and that those who are frail and different can only hope for a life worth living if we can find the right medication to change them back to being more like us. This causes us to devalue people who are differently abled and to hold lower expectations for people's well-being when our medical treatments do not solve the "problem." And as I mentioned earlier, well-being will never come out of a pill bottle.

McKnight and Block (2010) critique the "systems" approach created by a consumer-based society, including its effect on aging:

> Now old age is not even a category that is permissible on a death certificate. We now all die of a specific disease that we should have prevented through better living or detected sooner so that treatment would have worked. (p. 38)

Studies of people living with dementia show that, contrary to popular belief, quality of life does not necessarily decline, even with the progression of disability. Hopefully the examples and stories I have shared demonstrate that the assumption that a life without cure is a life of misery does not have to be the case in the majority of people, particularly if the harmful deficit-based social construct we have created around dementia can be replaced with one that supports well-being.

As we have discussed, much of that current construct results from the incredible stigma and fear that have been built around this illness, and the process of "othering" (Mitchell, DuPuis, & Kontos, 2013, p. 12) that it produces. DeBaggio (2002) once mused about stigmas when he noticed that a rat was stealing food pellets from his fish pond:

> Humans crave intimacy, and it is easily had with dogs, cats, birds, and fish. But a cantankerous rat, carrying the weight of centuries of hate and misunderstanding, becomes a target of fear. . . .
>
> What we do not understand, wild animal or human, we fear with murderous hate. . . . A disease like Alzheimer's has the same power to destroy as a bullet or scourge, through fear and misunderstanding . . . Now every morning I throw extra fish pellets into the lower pool for the rat. (p. 100)

In a remarkably prescient paper from 25 years ago (Lyman, 1989), the harmful social construct around dementia was referred to as the "medicalization of deviance." What are the larger implications for you and me when the time comes that we no longer match the appearance or abilities of the majority of adults? How will society treat us?

> The unfortunate byproduct of the belief in the discovery of a cure is that we have not begun thinking about ways that our society can see forgetfulness as something more than a demon to be exorcised by a hoped-for medical treatment. . . .
>
>   Yet, rather than a debilitating disease that leaves those afflicted in a sad and lamentable state of existence, dementia may be another, altered state of consciousness, as valuable and important as our everyday or "normal" way of being. This requires, foremost, a curiosity, an openness to all that is, to look at forgetfulness, as it is, not in the way we believe to know it. (Voris, Shabahangi, & Fox, 2009, pp. 119–120)

Mitchell et al. (2013) explain Olthuis's concept of knowing "otherwise" (Olthuis, 1997) as a practice of being with the person and accepting her reality for the insights and the greater potential for compassion it may provide. They propose that "knowing other-wise is an opportunity to see difference as potential wisdom instead of something to be changed or fixed" (p. 12).

It will always be difficult for individuals to live in a world of people who have a different level of cognitive ability. But while we look for treatments to slow the process of neuronal loss, we must also challenge our own views, assumptions, and prejudices that serve to reduce people with dementia to the sum of their broken parts, while ignoring the rich offerings and potential inherent in their emotional, spiritual, and relational selves.

As it stands now, the number of people living with dementia is expected to nearly triple by 2050. While I expect that we may discover new drug therapies to slow the progression of the illness, I do not expect that the total number of people living with these conditions will be dramatically less than our current predictions; that would only happen if an effective prevention or cure were developed, or if some other unexpected illness or event wiped out a large proportion of the older adult population. I believe policymakers need to accept the numbers as they are, and not hang their hopes on a significant reduction when setting goals for charting our future course.

So how do we plan for these coming demographic changes? By stepping back and looking at the larger issue of global aging. The stigmas surrounding dementia can be viewed as a part of the stigmas surrounding all older people. How we "think about" and respond to increasing numbers of people living with dementia represent a microcosm of how we will view and support the rapidly rising number of elders who we will see in the next few decades.

We can choose to bemoan the increasing number of older people, or we can discover ways in which our aging demographic can enrich our world and provide us with a sense of hope.

> The growing number of older people who expect health care and old age pensions should not be viewed as a threat or crisis. It is an opportunity, rather, to ensure decent living standards for all members of society, young and old, in the future. . . . It is the need to examine and make appropriate changes to health, social and economic policies, not the ageing of populations, that is the biggest challenge facing societies today. (World Health Organization, 1999, p. 20)

A perfect example of our societal blindness to this potential has been the branding of my (baby boomer) generation as "Generation Alzheimer's," based on the fact that our aging will produce more people living with Alzheimer's than ever before. Remember that the *incidence* of Alzheimer's is not rising over time for any given age group—in fact, some recently-published studies appear to support the notion that the age-specific incidence may well be falling. The rising total number of people with Alzheimer's simply reflects the mathematical fact that *my generation will produce more old people than ever before*. The proportion of U.S. adults 65 and older has grown from 4% in 1900 to 13% today, and will be closer to 20% by 2030.

But let us consider what these numbers also tell us: *there will also be more cognitively normal older people than ever before in our history*. So why are we not being called "Generation Cognitively Able"? My generation will also produce more 80-year-old CEOs and more 90-year-old marathon runners. There will be more elder volunteers in a variety of societal roles. There will be an unprecedented accumulation of life wisdom and experience—millions upon millions of new "historians." And the rising number of people with cognitive disorders also means there will be more people who can teach us the precepts of humanized care.

Finding hope in an aging population lies in focusing our attention on the strengths and possibilities rather than on the problems and deficits, so that we can imagine a different world in which we will grow old and possibly forgetful. So using the same strength-based approach that has framed this book, let us now craft a new vision for global aging, and then bring those living with dementia back into the center.

A New Vision for Aging

In *The World until Yesterday,* author Jared Diamond (2012) discusses how traditional and modern societies have treated their frail elders. In many traditional societies, a frail elder could become a liability, and as a result many were sacrificed for the overall survival of the tribe. That sacrifice ranged from abandonment, to assisted suicide, to outright murder by family members or other members of the tribe.

Diamond states, "We are fortunate that we do not face the same ordeal ourselves . . . because we have the good fortune to live in societies with surplus food and medical care" (p. 217). But maybe we are not as different as he postulates.

In traditional societies, there were two basic reasons for the tribe to consider abandoning or killing the old and frail: (1) having inadequate food or water to sustain all members of the tribe, or (2) needing to relocate the tribe quickly due to food shortage, weather extremes, or warfare, with frail elders who could not keep up.

Are there equivalents in our modern societies? Let us start with food shortages. Perhaps most industrialized countries have an adequate supply of food and water for their citizens; but what about other limited resources, such as available health care dollars? Will continued strains on our health care system due to an aging population force us to also deny resources to the most needy, in order to help the greater population survive?

And while modern nations are no longer nomadic, members of our society have been increasingly mobile in recent decades, such that younger generations tend to move farther from their parents than in centuries past. This means that the more traditional approach of living with one's elders as they age is all but extinct in many modern societies, as the younger members move on, leaving behind aging parents who "can't keep up" with their migrations. This removes an important social safety net for aging adults in modern societies. (To his credit, Diamond makes later statements that imply that these ironies were not lost on him.)

Diamond also makes the point that a major determinant of how much effort a tribe would expend to sustain its elders was their usefulness to the tribe. Once again, with the devaluation of older adults in our modern society, this yardstick does not bode well for aging baby boomers.

We may consider ourselves more civilized than traditional societies, and unlikely to force death on our elders even if society is burdened. But let us challenge this thought as well. When we consider that many frail elders are moved to nursing homes—many of which are very institutional and stifling—to end their days, and in many cases are rarely visited by relatives, if at all; when we consider that many hospitalization or insurance determinations are made based upon our societal idea of a person's potential; when we consider that neglect, abuse, and abandonment are far more common than we would like to believe; and when people such as the late Dr. Jack Kevorkian advocate for assisted suicide for those with dementia based on an expectation of intolerable suffering; we find that once again we are not all that different from the aboriginals who left their elders to the elements, or those who participated in assisted-suicide rituals.

Like our current deficit-based view of dementia, aging is seen as a disease that somehow must be stopped or seriously mitigated in order to create a healthy society. And like our biomedical approach to dementia, most of the proposed responses to global aging attempt to fix the problem, rather than shifting our paradigm and building on strengths.

The first step in our journey toward reframing and reclaiming hope is to create an attitude of inclusion, rather than exclusion. This will not only help create meaningful lives for older people in general, but will also help us to better address the needs of the increasing population who will experience cognitive shifts down the road.

In *Dementia Beyond Drugs*, I began with a critique of antipsychotic use to help burst the reader's bubble of belief in the value of these medications (which I termed the "pill paradigm"). To help shift the deficit-based "silver tsunami" paradigm, I will give a simple, pragmatic argument that shows how our current approach to segregating elders has been doomed from the start. The numbers have told us this for a long time, but we often do not see that which is right in front of us.

I could lay out a multitude of aging statistics to make my point, but the magnitude and volume of the numbers can be mind numbing. Perhaps the easiest way to drive my point home is with one statistic called the "potential support ratio" (PSR).

The PSR is an estimate of how many people are available to work and support those adults who are economically dependent. So the ratio is expressed as the number of people aged 15 to 64 for every adult aged 65 or older. Of course, some younger adults are unemployed, some older adults still work at jobs, and children are not included in this number.

Nevertheless, it gives us a rough estimate of the number of working adults for every retired adult.

In 1950, the global PSR was 12:1—that is, 12 working adults for every retired adult. By 2000, the ratio had dropped to 9:1, and by 2050, it is predicted to be only 4:1 (U.N. Report, 2011). So let us put aside any ethical issues for a moment and confront one fact: We cannot simply respond to an aging population by building more "senior communities" and nursing homes, because there will not be enough younger adults available to build or operate them!

Even if we engaged in drastic social engineering, such as significantly raising the retirement age, or closing all fast food restaurants and moving the employees to elder care careers, this number is inescapable. Our current practice of segregating older adults in society is doomed.

Beyond Segregation to the "Inclusive Society"

It should now be clear why I have continued to bring the argument against segregated "dementia care" to the forefront. A philosophy of inclusion holds insights for a new societal vision for aging. It is now time to craft this vision. Let us begin by imagining together a different possible future for our society, and then we will examine what needs to shift in order for us to realize this vision. We will use our processes of personal, operational, and physical transformation to take us to the Inclusive Society.

Our new society has undergone a transformation in our *personal* views of older adults and those living with dementia. We now see the value of older adults not only for what they can do, but also for *who they are*. This personal transformation comes from shifting three views that, according to Diamond (2012), have permeated modern society: (1) the work ethic, (2) the "cult of youth," and (3) the philosophy of individualism and self-reliance.

The work ethic is reflected in many common expressions, such as "putting one's nose to the grindstone" or "doing an honest day's labor." The value expressed is that applying oneself can create meaningful results, while laziness and lack of commitment to a task create a recipe for failure. The downside is that our work ethic has elevated productivity to the extent that those who cannot produce as much (due to various infirmities) are devalued, even if they have previously spent decades of their lives in highly productive work.

This ties closely into the cult of youth, as the young are generally healthier and stronger, and, therefore, can often produce more. Our society extols the value of those who work the most hours, score the most points on the athletic field, or take home the highest wages. At the same time, we actively devalue those at the other end of the spectrum. (Another example of this bias is the tendency of the well-to-do to blame the poor for their condition, often ignoring the subtle—or not-so-subtle—advantages that they have been handed by their upbringing, their race and social standing, or the many uncontrollable events, good or bad, in anyone's life.)

The new society we envision has shifted these two values to create a more balanced view. We now understand that there are more ways to contribute to the social fabric than through gainful employment. While these can involve being engaged in other forms of *doing*, they can also be expressed in the sharing of wisdom, experience, and perspective. Our aging boom is now an abundant source of both types of contributions.

In the realm of *doing*, one way in which retired adults contribute greatly to society is through volunteerism. This not only directly benefits the community, it also creates indirect economic benefits, because services are provided that do not require payment of salaries to others. Another form of volunteerism among older adults is grandparenting. As more households have dual working parents or single parents with children, the need for childcare becomes paramount. In 1999, it was estimated that there were "over 2 million children in the United States . . . being cared for by their grandparents, with 1.2 million of them living in their grandparents' home" (World Health Organization, 1999, p. 17). Grandparents have the added advantage of being well known to their grandchildren, thus strengthening familial bonds.

But in our new society, childcare does not need to occur purely among family members. We learned from communities such as the Iwate prefecture of Japan, where elders who are homebound are providing after-school care for the children of working neighbors in exchange for assistance with transportation or shopping. Older adults have time to be meaningfully "present" with children, and their ability to mentor the young has positive effects on their intellectual and social development. There is an economic savings to this type of arrangement in the short term; but the financial benefits that come about in the long term as the fabric of society strengthens through cooperation, trust, and collaboration reach beyond our ability to quantify.

Elders also possess much wisdom and experience that their younger counterparts do not have, simply by virtue of having lived longer. During the earthquake and tsunami that ravaged Ofunato, Japan, many people's lives were saved because the elders of the village recognized the danger signs and helped younger family members and neighbors understand the need to get to higher ground (HelpAge International, 2013). They were old enough to have experienced prior tsunamis and remembered the lessons of survival from those days. The elders of Ofunato who survived that day were also instrumental in helping the community to survive for an extended period of time without power or running water. They showed younger townspeople how to preserve food without electric refrigerators, cook without gas or electric stoves, and maintain sanitary conditions.

In communities unaffected by natural disaster, wisdom is shared in such ways as retired executives mentoring young businesspeople, or those who volunteer at places such as The Intergenerational School described in Chapter 8. The ways in which elders can share their wisdom with society are many, and our new society will more fully realize these contributions.

In *Dementia Beyond Drugs*, I described the work of the Macklin Intergenerational Institute, and the research showing that daily interactions with elders living with dementia significantly enhanced the personal and social development of preschool children. So the reintegration of those living with dementia into our society creates further benefits for the young.

And what about Diamond's third pervasive societal value of individualism and self-reliance? With apologies to Ralph Waldo Emerson, we have never been truly self-reliant. We have always benefited from the efforts of others, both vertically and horizontally. By "vertically," I mean that we stand on the shoulders of our forebears, our mentors, and those from generations past whom we never met, but whose wisdom forms the foundation for our own accomplishments. By "horizontally," I mean that we rely on our families, friends, co-workers, governments, and those who produce the various goods and services that we take for granted. "No man is an island. . . . "

Our new Inclusive Society has embraced this truth, and we temper our own achievements with the knowledge that our society is stronger and wiser when we support all of its constituents. We have now abandoned the all-or-none thinking about what elders, even frail elders, can contribute. Now we see older adults as more than—let's face it—parasites of our economic wealth, and we have learned how reciprocity can build both social and financial capital, creating a paradigm for successful global aging.

Here is another big shift we have made in our Inclusive Society, one which most policymakers and providers have not previously comprehended: *As long as we continue to view older people purely as consumers of services, global aging remains unaffordable and unsustainable in our current societal structure.*

We now see that our rush to simply increase "services" reflected a paternalistic attitude toward older people, and a blindness to what they also have to contribute. And this created excess disability, a population of "experts in the art of learning to need" (Illich, 1997, p. 23). This, in turn, added to our burdens and, as a consequence, the number of new services we needed to provide. We have now rejected what Robertson (1997) called the "commodification of need" (p. 429): one-way caregiving systems that, in effect, say "you are inadequate, incompetent, problematic, or broken. We will fix you. Go back to sleep" (McKnight & Block, 2010, p. 2).

We have now achieved a new paradigm that not only engages elders in reciprocal ways, but also reaches well beyond the realm of monetized arrangements. While many previous models for aging in community have helped to keep older residents engaged, most did so via a series of services for which the elders paid a fee. This kept life in the realm of consumerism and did not create the accountability that comes from a truly caring, trusting, and regenerative community. It also tended to perpetuate the one-way view of caregiving and did not see the potential of frail elders to add their talents to the community as we now see it.

A further shift in the community model was advanced with the concept of "time banking." Communities, recognizing that elders also have talents to offer, created a "barter system" of trading reciprocal benefits, such as providing after-school care or tutoring in return for transportation to shopping centers or appointments. However, we also learned not to put too much emphasis on the "equality" of these trades, knowing that expecting parity in all contributions does not value those who are able to do less, nor does it demonstrate our good commitment to look after our most vulnerable citizens.

Finally, our communities have responded to the increased separation of family members by creating engagement that reaches beyond family ties. This shift to a spirit of cooperation and openness has led to the empowerment and meaningful engagement of all community members, reducing excess disability and dependence. They have heeded the warnings of McKnight and Block (2010) that "the greatest tragedy of the consumer life is that its practitioners do not see that the local community is abundant with the relationships that are the principle resource for rescuing themselves and their families from failure, dependency, and isolation that are the results of a life as a consumer and client" (p. 18).

The reengagement of elders in our Inclusive Society has kept them from being "moved into the Third World—marginalized by the rest of society" (Gleckman, 2011). We have heard Margaret Mead's assertion from decades past that "if old people are separated from family life, there is real tragedy for them and the young." (Lustbader, 1991, p. 136)

Our Inclusive Society has combined the foregoing aspects of personal transformation with *physical* and *operational* transformations as well. We have abandoned the models of segregation that created not only dementia-specific housing, but also stand-alone nursing homes and other elder housing campuses, in favor of solutions that reintegrate those elders into the fabric of the larger community. For the most frail people who still require skilled care in congregate housing, small homes built on pioneering models such as the community Green House homes of St. John's in Rochester, New York, increasingly serve even the most frail among us within integrated, multigenerational communities.

And what of those community members who live with dementia? In Voris et al. (2009), Dr. Patrick Fox wonders:

> . . . can we create a world that is more "forgetfulness-friendly"?
>
> When you think of it in those terms, it's an idea that there are all kinds of ways of being that we accommodate for one reason or another. A good example is children born with Down syndrome. We create protective work environments and centers that cater to their needs. . . . But there are no pathways for dementia. . . . We think about it primarily in terms of a negative loss kind of mentality. (p. 110)

As you read these pages, a number of dementia-inclusive community initiatives are emerging around the world that seek to forge such pathways. These range from large-scale education and resource initiatives, such as those spearheaded by the U.K. Alzheimer's Society (http://www.alzheimers.org.uk/dementiafriendlycommunities), and Alzheimer's Australia (http://www.fightdementia.org.au/common/files/NAT/20130604_NAT_PUB_Paper31DementiaFriendlySocieties.pdf), to community-based projects such as York, England's, Dementia Without Walls, which is supported by the Joseph Rowntree Foundation (http://www.jrf.org.uk/publications/creating-dementia-friendly-york). Our new Inclusive Society has built on this work, and we have redesigned neighborhoods to accommodate our elders, adding such features as sidewalks, benches, ramps, and improved lighting and signage to our streets. We have expanded public transportation options and created satellite shops that bring basic necessities back within reach of most households. Community gardens, cafés (following the Ibasho Café model), and libraries provide other opportunities for elders to engage with their neighbors.

We have also educated our community members about how to communicate with and support our neighbors living with dementia, and we have provided opportunities for all citizens to continue to grow by engaging and participating with their neighborhoods and local businesses. And we have seen how powerful it is to learn as we go, to learn from each other, to collaborate, and to build on each success and each lesson learned.

But perhaps most important is that a commitment to inclusion has rendered previously invisible elders, of all abilities, visible in the social world again. Their participation has meant that our society is once again learning, as Rentsch (1997) suggests, "of the human meaning of finitude, the limitedness, and the vulnerability of man" (p. 271), and it has brought us closer to attaining "a consciousness of the value of slowness, of pausing, of calmly looking backward, of oral communication, of genuine conversation between real people and of being able to admit one was wrong" (p. 271).

"Two roads diverged in a yellow wood. . . ." (Robert Frost)

Which shall we choose?

Change is already happening, and it is up to us to craft the direction of these changes. If we do not begin to move toward the new Inclusive Society described throughout this chapter, the answers will be forced upon us in a more drastic, perhaps even violent, way, as our changing population overwhelms our inadequate approaches to aging and dementia.

How do we work together to move toward the Inclusive Society? On what do we focus? Where do we start? Bartlett and O'Connor (2010) eloquently sum up several key areas outlined in our new vision in their "social citizenship" approach to dementia (which are applicable to *all* older adults):

Principles underpinning a social citizenship approach:

- Active participation by people with dementia in their own lives, and society at large, must be maximised and valued.

- The potential for growth and positivity within the dementia experience must be recognised and promoted.

- Individual experiences and circumstances must be understood as inextricably connected to broader sociopolitical and cultural dynamics and structures.

- Solidarity between people with dementia, achieved through the fostering of a sense of "we" and community building, is a realistic goal that must be nurtured. (p. 70)

Later, they add that the "*UN research agenda on ageing for the 21st century*" identifies "care systems" as just one of the critical research arenas —it identifies nine others, including "*social participation and integration; economic security; macro-societal change and development; healthy ageing; quality of life; changing structures and functions of families, kin and community; and policy process and evaluation*" (p. 98).

This book outlines a pathway toward creating a society that values people whose cognition is different from that of the mainstream. It is a path to reducing excess disability and unnecessary drug use, thus easing the economic "burden" of these illnesses. It is a path to reconnecting people with each other and with meaningful lives, lives that can also benefit our larger society in meaningful ways.

It is also a path to reintegrating the difference and diversity that already exist in our communities, and to seeing the whole person, not simply the "disease." This approach can bring us together to create a healthier, more ethical, resilient, and inclusive society. In doing so, we will have a better opportunity to successfully meet the challenges that our world will face in the days ahead.

How might you be called upon to contribute?

And now, in order to take that first step along the pathway (as I advised at the start), I invite you to go back and read the Prologue one more time.

REFERENCES

Alonzo, T. (2013). Presentation on "Dementia care without drugs: A better approach" (with Anthony Chicotel) at the Alzheimer's Association Northern California and Northern Nevada Annual Education Conference, May 2, 2013, Sacramento, CA.

Aquilina, C., & Hughes, J.C. (2006). The return of the living dead: Agency lost and found? In J.C. Hughes, S.J. Luow, & S.R. Sabat (Eds.), *Dementia, mind, meaning and the person* (pp. 143–161). Oxford: Oxford University Press.

Arcare (2013). Internal corporate video on dedicated staffing process, filmed by Daniella Greenwood, culture strategy manager, Arcare Australia. www.arcare.com.au.

Arons, A.M.M., Krabbe, P.F.M., Schölzel-Dorenbos, C.J.M., van der Welt, G.J., & Olde Rikkert, M.G.M. (2013). Quality of life in dementia: A study of proxy bias. *BMC Medical Research Methodology, 13*, 110.

Baker, B. (2007). *Old age in a new age: The promise of transformative nursing homes.* Nashville: Vanderbilt University Press.

Ballard, C., Margallo-Lana, M., Theodoulou, M., Douglas, S., McShane, R., Jacoby, R., et al. (2008, April 1). A randomized, blinded, placebo-controlled trial in dementia patients continuing or stopping neuroleptics (The DART-AD Trial). Retrieved May 1, 2009 from PLoS Medicine web site: http://plosmedicine.org/article/info:doi/10.1371/journal.pmed.0050076.

Barrick, A.L., Rader, J., Hoeffer, B., Sloane, P.D., & Biddle, S. (2001). *Bathing without a battle: Person-directed care for individuals with dementia* (2nd ed.). New York: Springer.

Bartlett, R., & O'Connor, D. (2010). *Broadening the dementia debate: Towards social citizenship.* Bristol, U.K.: The Policy Press.

Behuniak, S.M. (2011). The living dead? The construction of people with Alzheimer's disease as zombies. *Aging & Society, 31*, 70–92.

Borrie, C. (2010). *The long hello.* Vancouver, BC: Nightwing Press.

Bowly, L. (2013). "To whom I may concern" produced by "A meeting of the minds" webinar series (www.mindsetmemory.com). Video can be viewed at: http://www.youtube.com/watch?v=PXn9AmFHGUM&feature=youtu.be.

Brady, C., & Frank, B. (2010). Presentation at Life Services Network annual conference, March 24–26, 2010, Chicago, IL.

Brilliant Image Productions. (2012). *20 questions, 100 answers, 6 perspectives* [DVD]. Available at www.brilliantimageproductions.com.

Bryden, C. (2011). Address at "A Changing Melody" conference, March 26, 2011, Toronto, Ontario, Canada.

Bryden, C. (2012). *Who will I be when I die?* (Originally published in 1998 under the name C. Boden). London: Jessica Kingsley Publishers.

Buettner, D. (2008). *The blue zones: Lessons for living longer from the people who've lived the longest.* Washington, DC: National Geographic.

Camp, C.J. (2012) *Hiding the stranger in the mirror: A detective's manual for solving problems associated with Alzheimer's disease and related disorders.* Solon, OH: Center for Applied Research in Dementia.

Carboni, J. (1990). Homelessness among the institutionalized elderly. *Journal of Gerontological Nursing, 16*(7), 3–37.

Carson, J. D. (2012). Presentation on "Liberating leisure in long-term care" at the 6th International Eden Alternative conference, May 30, 2012, Grand Rapids, MI.

Castle, N., & Anderson, R. (2011). Caregiver staffing in nursing homes and their influence on quality of care: Using dynamic panel estimation methods. *Medical Care, 49*(6), 545–552.

Clare, L., Rowlands, J., & Quin, R. (2008). Collective strength: The impact of a shared social identity in early-stage dementia. *Dementia 7*, 9–30.

Cochrane Report. (2012). There is limited evidence to support the assumption that the care of people with dementia in special care units is superior to care in traditional nursing units. Published online May 16, 2012, at http://summaries.cochrane.org/CD006470/.

Davis, R. (1989). *My journey into Alzheimer's disease: Helpful insights for family and friends.* Carol Stream, IL: Tyndale House.

Dean, D. (2007). *The Madonnas of Leningrad.* New York: Harper Perennial.

DeBaggio, T. (2002). *Losing my mind: An intimate look at life with Alzheimer's.* New York: The Free Press.

DeBaggio, T. (2003). *When it gets dark: An enlightened reflection on life with Alzheimer's.* New York: The Free Press

Dessel, R., & Ramirez, M. (2013a). *Policies and procedures concerning sexual expression at the Hebrew Home at Riverdale.* Sexual expression policy. Available at the Home's web site: http://www.hebrewhome.org/uploads/ckeditor/files/sexualexpressionpolicy.pdf.

Dessel, R., & Ramirez, M. (2013b). *Policies and procedures concerning sexual expression at the Hebrew Home at Riverdale.* Sexual consent guidelines. Available at the home's website: http://www.hebrewhome.org/uploads/ckeditor/files/sexualconsentguidelines.pdf.

Devanand, D.P., Mintzer, J., Schultz, S.K., Andrews, H.F., Sultzer, D.L., de la Pena, D., et al. (2012). Relapse risk after discontinuation of risperidone in Alzheimer's disease. *New England Journal of Medicine, 367*(16), 1497–1507.

Diamond, J. (2012). *The world until yesterday: What can we learn from traditional societies?* New York: Penguin Group.

Digh, P. (2008). *Life is a verb: 37 days to wake up, be mindful, and live intentionally.* Guilford, CT: Skirt.

DuPuis, S.L., Gillies, J., Carson, J., Whyte, C., Genoe, R., Loiselle, L., & Sadler, L. (2012). Moving beyond 'patient' and 'client' approaches: Mobilising authentic partnerships in dementia care. *Dementia: The International Journal of Social Research and Practice, 11*(4), 427–452.

Dupuis, S.L., Whyte, C., & Carson, J. (2012). Leisure in long-term care settings. In J. Singleton & H. Gibson (Eds.), *Leisure and aging: Theory and practice.* Champaign, IL: Human Kinetics.

Dupuis, S.L., Whyte, C., Carson, J., Genoe, R., Meshino, L., & Sadler, L. (2012). Just dance with me: An authentic partnership approach to understanding leisure in the dementia context. *World Leisure Journal, 54*(3), 240–254.

Edvardsson, D., Winblad, B., & Sandman, P. O. (2008). Person-centred care of people with severe Alzheimer's disease: Current status and way forward. *Lancet Neurol, 7*, 362–367.

Eliopoulos, C. (2010). *Invitation to holistic health: A guide to living a balanced life* (2nd ed.). Burlington, MA: Jones and Bartlett.

Farrell, D., & Frank, B. (2007). A keystone for excellence: Implementing consistent assignment provides a string foundation for achieving goals of the Advancing Excellence in America's Nursing Homes program. *Provider* (July), 35–38.

Fazio, S. (2008). *The enduring self in people with Alzheimer's: Getting to the heart of individualized care.* Baltimore: Health Professions Press.

Feil, N. (2002). *The validation breakthrough.* Baltimore: Health Professions Press.

Fick, D., Kolanowski, A., & Waller, J. (2007). High prevalence of central nervous system medications in community-dwelling adults with dementia over a three-year period. *Aging and Mental Health, 11*(5), 588–595.

Fossey, J., Ballard, C., Juszczak, E., James, I., Alder, N., Jacoby, R., et al. (2006). Effect of enhanced psychosocial care on antipsychotic use in nursing home residents with severe dementia: Cluster randomized trial. *British Medical Journal, 332,* 756–761.

Fox, N. (1995). Postmodern perspectives on care: The vigil and the gift. *Critical Social Policy, 15,* 107–125.

Fox, N., Norton, L., Rashap, A.W., Angelelli, J., Tellis-Nayak, V., et al. (2005). Well-being: Beyond quality of life [white paper]. Now available as "The Eden Alternative Domains of Well-Being™: Revolutionizing the Experience of Home by Bringing Well-Being to Life," at www.edenalt.org.

Frankl, V. (1959). *Man's search for meaning.* New York: Simon & Schuster.

George, D., & Whitehouse, P. (2011). Marketplace of memory: What the brain fitness technology industry says about us and how we can do better. *Gerontologist, 51*(5), 590–596.

Gleckman, H. (2011). Walter Mosley on becoming marginalized in old age. In *Forbes* online: http://www.forbes.com/sites/howardgleckman/2011/12/02/walter-mosley-on-becoming-marginalized-in-old-age/.

Greenblat, C. (2011). *Love, loss, and laughter: Seeing Alzheimer's differently.* Guilford, CT: Lyons Press.

Greenwood, D. (2012). Arcare: A relational approach to building a dementia strategy [internal document].

Guildermann, S.A., Jaeger, M., & Morris, C. (2013). Presentation on "Falling into culture change: A blueprint for a fall prevention program" at the Pioneer Network National Conference, August 12, 2013, Bellevue, WA.

Haralabidas, A.S., Dimakopoulou, K., Vigna-Taglianti, F., Giampaolo, M., Borgini, A., Dudley, M.-L., et al. (2008). Acute effects of night-time noise exposure on blood pressure in populations living near airports. *European Heart Journal, 129,* 658–664.

HelpAge International (2013). Displacement and older people: The case of the great east Japan earthquake and tsunami in 2011. Report available at www.helpage.org.

Henderson, C. S. (1998). *Partial view: An Alzheimer's journal.* Dallas: Southern Methodist University Press.

Hoe, J., Hancock, G., Livingston, G., & Orrell, M. (2006). Quality of life of people with dementia in residential care homes. *British Journal of Psychiatry, 188,* 460–464.

Howorth, M., Keady, J., Riley, G., & Drummond, G. (2012). The Open Doors network: Dementia and self-growth. *British Journal of Mental Health Nursing, 1*(2), 38–41.

Illich, I. (1977). Disabling professions. In Illich, I., Zola, I. K., McKnight, J., Caplan, J., and Shaiken, H. (Eds.), *Disabling professions.* London: Marion Boyers.

Kitwood, T. (1997). *Dementia reconsidered: The person comes first.* New York: Open University Press.

Kitwood, Y., & Bredin, K. (1992). Towards a theory of dementia care: personhood and well-being. *Aging and Society, 12,* 269–287.

Kiyota, E. (2011). Presentation at St. John's Home in Rochester, NY, May 25, 2011.

Kunik, M.E., Snow, A.L., Davila, J.A., Steele, J.B., Balasubramanyam, V., Doody, R. S., et al. (2010). Causes of aggressive behavior in patients with dementia. *Journal of Clinical Psychiatry, 71*(9), 1145–1152.

Lustbader, W. (1991) *Counting on kindness: The dilemmas of dependency.* New York: The Free Press.

Lyman, K.A. (1989). Bringing the social back in: A critique of the biomedicalization of dementia. *The Gerontologist, 29*(5), 597–605.

Maslow, A.H. (1943). A theory of human motivation. *Psychological Review, 50*, 370–396.

Max-Neef, M., Elizade, A., & Hopenhayn, M. (1991). Development in human needs. In Max-Neef, M. (Ed.), *Human scale development: Conception, application, and further reflections*. London: The Apex Press, pp. 13–54.

McGowin, D.F. (1993). *Living in the labyrinth: A personal journey through the maze of Alzheimer's*. New York: Dell.

McKnight, J., & Block, P. (2010). *The abundant community: Awakening the power of families and neighborhoods*. San Francisco: Barrett-Kohler.

McLean, A. (2007). Dementia care as a moral enterprise: A call for a return to the sanctity of lived time. *Alzheimer's Care Today* (formerly, *Alzheimer's Care Quarterly*), 8(4), 360–372.

Mitchell, G.J., DuPuis, S.L., & Kontos, P.C. (2013). Dementia discourse: From imposed suffering to knowing *other-wise*. *Journal of Applied Hermeneutics*, June 12, Article 5, 1–19.

Morgan, R.O., Sail, K.R., Snow, A.L., Davila, J.A., Fouladi, N.N., & Kunik, M.E. (2013). Modeling causes of aggressive behavior in patients with dementia. *The Gerontologist*, 53(5), 738–747.

Nolan, M.R., Brown, J., Davies, S., Nolan, J., & Keady, J. (2006). *The Senses Framework: Improving care for older people through a relationship-centred approach*. Getting Research into Practice (GRiP) Report No 2. Project Report. University of Sheffield. Available at: http://shura.shu.ac.uk/id/eprint/280.

Nouwen, H.J.M. (2004). *Out of solitude: Three meditations on the Christian life*. Notre Dam, IN: Ave Maria Press.

Nygard, K. (2012) Presentation at symposium, "Unleash the power of person-directed care," Nashville, Tennessee, December 3, 2012.

O'Connor, D. (2002). Toward empowerment: ReVisioning family support groups. *Social Work with Groups*, 25(4), 37–56.

Olthuis, J.H. (Ed.). (1997). *Knowing other-wise: Philosophy at the threshold of spirituality*. New York: Fordham University Press.

Pearce, N. (2011). *Inside Alzheimer's: How to hear and honor connections with a person who has dementia* (revised edition). Taylors, SC: Forrason Press.

Pedlar, A., Hornbrook, T., & Haasen, B. (2001). Patient-focused care: Theory and practice. *Therapeutic Recreation Journal*, 35(1), 15–30.

Power, G.A. (2010). *Dementia beyond drugs: Changing the culture of care*. Baltimore: Health Professions Press.

Power, G.A. (2012a). Dementia doesn't cause "sundowning"—we do. *Journal of Dementia Care*. 20(3), 15.

Power, G.A. (2012b). Should we drop "dementia" from the DSM-V? [blog post] Available at: http://changingaging.org/alpower/2012/11/29/should-we-drop-dementia-from-the-dsm-5/.

Rentsch, T. (1997). Aging as becoming oneself: A philosophical ethics of late life. *Journal of Aging Studies*, 11(4), 263–271.

Rhee, Y.J., Csernansky, J.G., Emanuel, L.L., Chang, C.G., & Shega, J.W. (2011). Psychotropic medication burden and factors associated with antipsychotic use. *Journal of the American Geriatric Society*, 59(11), 2100–2107.

Robertson, A. (1997). Beyond apocalyptic demography: Towards a moral economy of interdependence. *Aging and Society*, 17, 425–446.

Rose, L. (2003). *Larry's way: Another look at Alzheimer's from the inside*. New York: iUniverse.

Sabat, S.R., Johnson, A., Swarbrick, C., & Keady, J. (2011). The "demented other" or simply "a person"? Extending the philosophical discourse of Naue and Kroll through the situated self. *Nursing Philosophy, 12,* 282–292.

SACFER (Southeast Advocacy Center for Elder Rights). (2012). *Survival manual for elders: Encouraging elders' resiliency potential.* Walden, TN: Waldenhouse Publishers.

Sacks, O. (2012). *Hallucinations.* New York: Alfred A. Knopf.

Sands, L.P., Ferreira, P., Stewart, A.L., Brod, M., & Yaffe, K. (2004). What explains differences between dementia patients' and their caregivers' ratings of patients' quality of life? *American Journal of Geriatric Psychiatry, 12*(3), 272–280.

Schmidt, F.P., Basner, M., Kröger, G., Weck, S., Schnorbus, B., Muttray, A., et al. (2013). Effect of nighttime aircraft noise exposure on endothelial function and stress hormone release in healthy adults. *European Heart Journal, 34*(45), 3508–3514.

Schrjvers, E.M., Verhaaren, B.F., Koudstaal, P.J., Hofman, A., Ikram, M.A., & Breteler, M. M. (2012). Is dementia incidence declining? Trends in dementia incidence since 1990 in the Rotterdam Study. *Neurology, 78*(19), 1456–1463.

Shabahangi, N.R., & Szymkiewicz, B. (2008). *Deeper into the soul: Beyond dementia and Alzheimer's toward forgetfulness care.* San Francisco: Elders Academy Press.

Shabahangi, N. (2014). Chapter 16: Humanistic eldercare: Toward a new conceptual framework for aging. In Schneider, K.J., Pierson, J.F., & Bugental, J.F.T. (Eds.), *The handbook of humanistic psychology* (2nd edition). Thousand Oaks, CA: Sage Publications, pp. 213–226.

Shanks, L.K. (1999). *Your name is Hughes Hannibal Shanks: A caregiver's guide to Alzheimer's.* Lincoln: University of Nebraska Press.

Shouse, D. (2006). *Love in the land of dementia: Finding hope in the caregiver's journey.* Kansas City, MO: The Creativity Connection Press.

Simpson, R., & Simpson, A. (1999). *Through the wilderness of Alzheimer's: A guide in two voices.* Minneapolis: Augsburg.

Sinclair, U. (1935). *I, Candidate for Governor: And how I got licked.* Reprint 1994. Berkeley: University of California Press.

Spector, W.D., Limcango, R., Williams, C., Rhodes, W., & Hurd, D. (2013). Potentially avoidable hospitalizations for elderly long-stay residents in nursing homes. *Medical Care, 51*(8), 673–681.

Sturm, V.E., Yokoyama, J.S., Seeley, W.W., Kramer, J.H., Miller, B.L., & Rankin, K.P. (2013). Heightened emotional contagion in mild cognitive impairment and Alzheimer's disease is associated with temporal lobe degeneration. *Proceedings of the National Academy of Sciences USA, 110*(24), 9944–9949.

Swain, J., French, S., & Cameron, C. (2003). *Controversial issues in a disabling society.* Buckingham: Open University Press.

Sylvester, C. (1987). Therapeutic recreation and the end of leisure. *Philosophy of Therapeutic Recreation, 1,* 76–89.

Taylor, R. (2007). *Alzheimer's from the inside out.* Baltimore: Health Professions Press.

Taylor, R. (2012). "Hello Dinner" [DVD]. *Dementia Support Network, USA.* Available at: http://www.richardtaylorphd.com/free-stuff/2012-05-21-16-16-52.html.

Taylor, R. (2011). Presentation at St. John's Home in Rochester, NY, February 9, 2011.

Thomas, W.H. (2004). *What are old people for? How elders will save the world.* Acton, MA: VanderWyk & Burnham.

Thomas, W. H. (2012). Panel discussion on surplus safety at the 6th Eden International Conference, May 30–June 1, 2012, Grand Rapids, Michigan.

UN Report: Department of Economic and Social Affairs. (2011). *World population ageing: 1950–2050.* Available at: http://www.un.org/esa/population/publications/world ageing19502050/.

Verity, J. (2010). Presentation of "The *Spark of Life* Approach" at St. John's Home in Rochester, New York, June 10, 2010.

Verity, J., & Lee, H. (2008). *Spark of Life club program handbook. A whole new world of dementia care.* Mooroolbark, Victoria, Australia: Dementia Care Australia Pty. Ltd.

Vonnegut, K. (1969). *Slaughterhouse—Five.* Reprint 1991. New York: Dell.

Voris, E., Shabahangi, N., & Fox, P. (2009). *Conversations with Ed: Waiting for forgetfulness: Why are we so afraid of Alzheimer's disease?* San Francisco: Elders Academy Press.

Whitehouse, P.J., & George, D. (2008). *The myth of Alzheimer's: What you aren't being told about today's most dreaded condition.* New York: St. Martin's.

Wong, C.K. (2009). *Even when she forgot my name: Love, life and my mother's Alzheimer's.* Singapore: Epigram.

World Health Organization (WHO). (1999). Ageing: Exploding the myths. Geneva: WHO. Available at: http://whqlibdoc.who.int/hq/1999/who_hsc_ahe_99.1.pdf.

Zeisel, J., Silverstein, N.M., Hyde, J., Levkoff, S., Lawton, M.P., & Holmes, W. (2003). Environmental correlates to behavioral health outcomes in Alzheimer's special care units. *The Gerontologist, 43*(5), 697–711.

RESOURCES

20 Questions, 100 Answers, 6 Perspectives DVD (Brilliant Image Productions) http://www.bestdementiavideosandbooks.com

Alive Inside (film) http://aliveinside.us

Alzheimer's Association (U.S.) http://www.alz.org

Alzheimer's Disease International (ADI) http://www.alz.co.uk

Alzheimer's Foundation of America http://www.alzfdn.org

Arcare Aged Care http://www.arcare.com.au

ARTZ (Artists for Alzheimer's) http://www.artistsforalzheimers.org

By Us For Us Guides http://www.uwaterloo.ca/murray-alzheimer-research-and-education-program/education-and-knowledge-translation/products-education-tools/by-us-for-us-guides

ChangingAging (Allen Power's blog) http://www.changingaging.org/alpower

Dementia Action Alliance (U.K.) http://www.dementiaaction.org.uk

Dementia Action Alliance (U.S.) http://www.ccal.org/the-dementia-action-alliance/

Dementia Advocacy and Support Network International http://www.dasninternational.org

Dementia Support Networks (U.S.) http://www.richardtaylorphd.com/free-stuff/2012-05-21-16-16-52.html

The Eden Alternative® http://www.edenalt.org

The Eden Alternative Domains of Well-Being™ white paper http://www.edenalt.org/images/stories/tools_for_registery/EdenWell-BeingWhitePaperv5.pdf

The Green House® Project http://www.thegreenhouseproject.org

Hello Dinners http://www.richardtaylorphd.com/component/content/article/55-dementia-support-networks/74-hello-dinners.html

Ibasho http://www.ibasho.org

I Can! I Will! http://www.alz.co.uk/icaniwill

The Intergenerational Schools (Cleveland, OH) http://www.tisonline.org/tis/

IN2L http://www.in2l.com

LifeBio http://www.lifebio.com

Murray Alzheimer Research and Education Program (MAREP) http://www.uwaterloo.ca/murray-alzheimer-research-and-education-program/

A Meeting of the Minds http://www.minds-meeting.com

Music and Memory http://www.musicandmemory.org

National Dementia Initiative white paper http://www.ccal.org/national-dementia-initiative/white-paper/

Pacific Institute http://www.pacificinstitute.org

Pioneer Network http://www.pioneernetwork.net

Richard Taylor's blog http://www.richardtaylorphd.com/blog.html

St. John's Home and Green House Homes (Rochester, NY) http://www.stjohnsliving.org

TimeSlips http://www.timeslips.org

UK Dementia Congress http://www.careinfo.org/

UK *Journal of Dementia Care* http://www.careinfo.org/journal-of-dementia-care/

INDEX

Note: *f* indicates figures.

Acare (Australia), 87–90
Acetylcholine, 203
Acoustic environment
  anxiety and, 107
  auditing, 133–134
  autonomy and, 145, 167
  music in, 52–53, 240–241, 245–248,
    252–263
Activity programming
  assessment and, 177, 180, 189
  for brain fitness, 223–224
  security and, 132
  shortcomings of, 176, 177–178,
    181–182
  well-being and, 28–30, 29*f*
Admission process, 53–55, 56
Adult day programs, 181, 216–217
Advocacy, 28–30, 29*f*, 150, 192–193
Ageism, 128, 138–139, 141
Aggression, *see* Behavioral expressions
    of dementia
Aging
  Alzheimer's disease and, 272
  growth and, 217
  identity and, 45
  new vision for, 276–278
  in place, 45
  systems approach and, 273
Aging in place, 45
Agitation, 108–110, 211–212
  see also Restlessness
Airline passenger stories, 139, 142
Alarms
  for beds/chairs, 106–107, 126
  limiting physical space and, 114–115
  removal at exits, 126–127
  risk and, 97, 107–108
Alienation/separation, 65
Alive Inside (film), 52
All-or-none thinking, 116–117, 151
Alzheimer's disease
  future of, 270–276
  joy and, 235–236
  personhood and, 232

research/education program, 28–30,
    29*f*, 192–193
  security and, 128
  senses and, 240, 241–242
  stigma and, 68
  stories, *see* Alzheimer's disease stories
Alzheimer's disease stories
  autonomy, 148–149, 151, 158,
    159–160
  connectedness, 65, 79 68–69, 243,
    273
  growth, 209, 215–217, 218, 219,
    221–222, 228–229
  identity, 39
  meaning, 182
  security, 113
"Amazing Grace" story, 245–248
Anti-Parkinson drugs, 204
Antipsychotic drugs
  in community based-living, 15–16
  emotional expression and, 143
  evidence on, 17–18, 203–204, 209
  stories, 122–123
  well-being framework and, 254
Anxiety
  body language and, 199
  connectedness and, 92
  death and, 182
  posttraumatic stress, 113–114
  questioning and, 153
  security and, 101, 107, 108, 110, 120
Artists for Alzheimer's (ARTZ), 240
ARTZ (Artists for Alzheimer's), 240
Assessment
  activities/leisure and, 177, 180, 189
  at admissions, 54, 56
  growth and, 209–210
  identity and, 43
  of strengths vs. deficits, 215
Assisted living
  autonomy and, 144, 170
  connectedness and, 79–80
  integrated care and, 214
  meaning and, 185–186, 187
  stories, 60–61, 113–115, 216
Audits, 133–134, 252